Stress Management

Stress Management

A Manual for Nurses

Vicki D. Lachman, R.N., Ph.D.

V. L. Associates
Philadelphia, Pennsylvania

W.B. SAUNDERS COMPANY
Harcourt Brace Jovanovich, Inc.
Philadelphia London Toronto Montreal Sydney Tokyo

Library of Congress Cataloging-in-Publication Data

Lachman, Vicki D.
    Stress management.

    Bibliography: p.
    Includes index.
    1. Nursing—Psychological aspects.   2. Nurses—Job
stress.   3. Nurses—Mental health.   4. Burn-out
(Psychology)   I. Title.   [DNLM: 1. Stress, Psychological
—Prevention and control—Nursing texts.   2. Nursing.
WY 16 L138s]
RT86.L33   1983   610'.73'06'9   83-10783
ISBN 0-8089-1554-1

Library of Congress Catalog Number 83-10783
International Standard Book Number 0-8089-1554-1

Printed in the United States of America
85 86 87 88   10 9 8 7 6 5 4 3 2

Special thanks to

Suzanne Hall-Johnson, who gave me the courage to write

Carol Wolfe, who gave me the chance
to publish this book

Regina Thorell, who gave me hours of her time typing
and retyping this manuscript

my friends, who gave me encouragement, understanding,
and patience to complete this book

*This book is dedicated to you and all nurses—
nurses who each day run some cog
in the wheel of the health care system.*

Contents

CHAPTER 1.

Stress and Burnout Phenomena: Clarifying the Issue   1

Case Histories: Who Is Being Affected?
    Practitioner
    Educator
    Manager
Definition of the Problem: What Is Burnout?

CHAPTER 2.

Physical Strategies: Protecting Your Body   17

Lifestyle Habits Can Create Illness
How the Body Handles Stress
Heredity and Family Attitude
Physical Signs and Symptoms of Stress
Environmental Conditions and Lifestyle Factors
Methods of Stress Reduction
    Muscle relaxation and tension release techniques
    Progressive relaxation and visual imagery
    Meditation and breathing
    Physical fitness
    Diversion
Prevention Tactics
    Wellness philosophy
    Health risk appraisals

Contents

List of Assessments

Chapter 6   Management

Chapter 7   Change

Chapter 8   Planning

Foreword

Job stress is not unique to nursing. Burnout is a common syndrome in many professions, including teaching and engineering, and some professionals find it even harder to cope with job stress than do nurses.

Nursing, however, possesses a unique pattern of stress. The strains rooted in the conflicts of the changing role of women, the pressures for cost-effectiveness in health care, and disagreements on what the nurse does all result in a unique pattern of job stress. Nurses, while exerting their own expertise and independence, have to deal with others who expect them to do what they are told. They are expected to get more work done, more efficiently, and often with less staff in order to reduce the cost of health care. Finally, nurses must deal with the role conflicts engendered by others' expectations, since there is wide diversity of opinion within and without the nursing profession as to what the nurse should do.

This book offers welcome solutions to the problem of stress management for nurses. Although other books have dealt with burnout and the presence of stress in nursing, this book hits, for the first time, the critical issue in stress management: the importance of the individual nurse. Although stress management is a professional problem, it must be confronted and handled by each nurse individually. The author has included many personal activities in each section where nurses can find help in managing their particular conflicts, whether they are in clinical, educational, or management positions.

In addition, the book clearly identifies the significant goal of stress management: increased enjoyment of nurses in their work. Past literature focused more on the length of time the nurse spent in nursing than on personal and professional enjoyment of that work, but this text discusses both building self-esteem and increasing enjoyment at work.

Finally, this book truly focuses on stress management, per se; that is, it goes beyond describing the stressors to show how to handle the problems that arise from job stress. Specific techniques are clearly described, including building stress tolerance, preventing stress, changing addictions, and developing individual stress management programs. The author encourages readers to develop their own stress management techniques tailored to their needs and based on level of work stress, expertise, and personality.

This book is, as all books are, a reflection of the author who conceived the idea and toiled through the writing. Vicki Lachman brings much of her personal and professional self to you in these pages. She has truly mastered the art of handling stressors in nursing, not in only one setting but in many clinical, management, and educational positions in both private and public agencies. Her personal excitement and professional enjoyment are apparent in the strategies presented here in *Stress Management: A Manual For Nurses.*

Suzanne Hall Johnson, R.N., M.N.
Director, Health Update
Editor, *Dimensions of Critical Care Nursing*

Preface

The answer to why this book was written is best begun with a brief story that spans the last 19 years (1964–1983). During these years as a staff nurse, evening charge nurse, night supervisor, clinical specialist, nurse educator, and nurse in private practice, I watched how people take care of their health—and became increasingly curious as to what kept some people healthier than others. According to the research reported by Pines (1980), stress-resistant people, the healthy people, have a set of attitudes toward life: they exhibit an openness to change, a feeling of involvement in whatever they are doing, and a sense of control over events. Put another way, they score high on measures of challenge, commitment, and control.

A 40-year prospective study by Valliant (1979) showed interesting results on the use of defense mechanisms to stay healthy. The four adaptation mechanisms seen as desirable were humor, altruism, sublimination, and suppression. Even when the contributions of smoking, suicide, alcohol use, obesity, and age of death of parents and grandparents had been controlled for, the correlation between the mode of defense and physical health remained significant.

In contemplating these results I began a project to study what keeps *nurses* healthy. This project became the substance for this book, my doctoral dissertation, and stress management workshops I do throughout the country. Having read over 200 articles and 40 books on stress and burnout, as well as talked to hundreds of nurses, I have come to realize that some key problems exist in an individual's ability to manage personal and professional stress. The conclusions repeatedly point to the fact that stress is manageable when one practices a healthy lifestyle, feels successful and satisfied in work and relationships, and learns to deal with the changes of life.

The events during this almost 20-year span of time in our world have made the stress of change more difficult to manage. The individual in this century is faced with demands requiring decisions that affect both physical and emotional health. These decisions must be informed ones; they will affect the quality of the individual's life for years to come. Additionally, nursing has been profoundly affected with the expanding health care system, women's liberation, and the information explosion. Specifically, the effects of the physician's assistant, unprepared nursing managers, and the increased complexity of patient care are still not realized. Nursing, like other health professions, was not prepared for the continuing need to adjust to increasing and rapid changes. This stress of change in the personal and professional spheres is affecting both nurses' health and the health of the nursing profession.

Learning the skills to cope with change and to create some of one's own changes can do wonders to decrease the stress level. This manual is designed to teach these skills. It will help one ask the questions one needs to ask in order to be able to make health-promoting decisions while dealing with the stress in both personal and professional life.

Demands are continually placed upon nurses to act responsibly; people are their responsibility. They are held accountable for quality patient care, quality education, and the effective management of nursing personnel. Many times they are expected to perform these functions without adequate resources, without the needed authority that goes with the responsibility, and finally without the commensurate rewards.

This manual is designed to help nurses improve their careers so that the responsibilities and the problems don't drive them out. Several chapters are focused directly on the work climate. Others address skills needed to function effectively and happily in their careers and homes.

Some stresses are inherent in nursing. Other sources of stress originate from the problems in the health care and health education system—these problems can and should be solved. This manual was created to act as a resource to help nurses cope with the inherent stresses and to give them some of the skills to begin to change the system in which nurses work. The goal is a qualitatively better professional life.

This book is for the individual practicing nurse, nurse educator, and nurse manager interested in improving the quality of his or her work life. Individuals can use the book as a personal stress management workbook—reading the information, answering the questions, and contemplating and designing a personal stress control program. I suggest reading this manual with a pencil and pad at hand. For the most effective use of this book readers will need to take the self-assessment questionnaires presented throughout the text. No matter what your function in nursing, you will benefit from increasing your repertoire of stress coping methods.

Nurse educators can use the manual as a course guide for a stress management course. It covers the aspects I teach in my 16-hour course, although in much more depth. The book chapters could also act as a discussion guide for a course or a support group.

The beginning chapter is meant to introduce you to the concepts of stress and burnout through case studies of nurses I have treated or talked with over the years. May their familiar-sounding nature guide you to continue, to see how burnout doesn't have to be inevitable for you. Burnout is a preventable syndrome. By following the guides in the chapters, practicing the techniques, and utilizing the strategies outlined, you can manage your stress.

In Chapter 2 the focus is on developing your resistance to stress by creating a physically fit body and a relaxed mind. While recognizing that you cannot prevent all stress, you will need to develop ways to help your body and mind cope with negative stress consequences. Exercise rids the body of excess catecholamines, and relaxation methods give you nonthinking time to reduce mental tension. Other holistic methods of achieving a resilient body are mentioned.

Your cognitive appraisal of events plays a large role in determining your level of stress. By viewing stressful events as challenging rather than threatening you are more likely to transform these events to your advantage. If you try to deny these situations by drinking too much, taking drugs, or sleeping more, you are likely to end up in endless rumination and preoccupation. As anyone who has ever used some of these tactics to deal with problems can attest, the problem does not go away. The source of stress remains and continues to exert its effects.

Chapter 3 focuses on developing a cognitive set that promotes an attitude of dealing with life's challenges. The premise of this chapter is based on the ideas of Lazarus (1966), who emphasized that stress resides neither in the person nor in the situation alone, but depends on how the person appraises particular events. The mechanism that produces a stress-related illness has been presumably physiological. Personality traits such as viewing change as a challenge, however, may be more important than was once thought.

Chapter 4, on the other hand, is designed to help you see that some habits may be unconscious mechanisms for coping with stress. Smoking, drugs, and overeating are all ways to temporarily reduce stress levels; each distracts from approaching the life stress directly. Therefore recommendations abound in this chapter on how to recognize and change addictive coping patterns.

In Chapter 5 the purpose is to tune you into identifying the key factors affecting your work satisfaction. Methods of assessing your work climate are numerous. Ideas to increase job satisfaction are focused on decreasing the source of stress or on changing your approach to the stressor. "Choosing Your Best Career Path" concludes this chapter with a focus on the three key aspects for a satisfying career.

Since most nurses were not taught to understand their organizational system, Chapter 6 affords the nurse the opportunity to look at the organizational climate of the institution. Examples of what some organizations are doing to reduce the stress in nursing are given. The chapter ends by exploring the four key management skills.

Managers, please note especially Chapters 5 and 6, since they are relevant to improving the work climate of your staff. As a manager you may also be responsible for the selection of a stress management course, and the book is meant to guide you in the selection of course content. You will learn which issues are especially important to address and you will begin to develop management level strategies to reduce the stress of your staff to increasingly tolerable levels.

In the final two chapters the focus is on dealing with change and making health promotion changes. Certain skills, such as goal setting and time management, help make adaptation to externally or internally generated changes easier. Chapter 8 guides you in developing a step-by-step approach to designing your personal stress reduction change.

From start to finish the purpose of this book is to guide you in reducing your stress to a level that is comfortable and healthy for you. In its three-year creation this manual has been a constant reminder that I can manage stress. My hope is that this book will help you take care of yourself while taking care of others.

Stress
Management

1

Stress and Burnout Phenomena: Clarifying the Issue

Professional nurses in the fields of clinical practice, management, and education are affected by stress directly and indirectly. Some of the stories that follow may sound autobiographical to you. Some may create images of your past experience in nursing, and others may reflect what you hope not to feel in the future.

Allow me to introduce you to three nurses whose problems may be very familiar to you. As you read their histories imagine the stress they feel. After considering these examples you will be better able to understand the causes of burnout.

Practitioner

Mary Alice, a staff nurse, is the charge nurse of a 40-bed medical unit in a metropolitan hospital. The unit is very active, and many of the patients require detailed nursing care. Short staffed and unable to provide good-quality nursing care, Mary often feels guilty, as does the rest of the staff. She often wonders if people really understand that the nurses are doing the best they can, considering the circumstances they have to work under. "The four chief physicians servicing this area are all test happy," says Mary Alice. "Multiple lab tests and x-rays on the daily activities schedule is S.O.P. Patients complain to us every day, as if we ordered the test."

Two of the medical doctors are frequently cited by the staff as being critical, demanding physicians. They create an environment that is always

1

potentially explosive. Mary Alice occasionally blows up at one of them after "having taken it long enough."

The hospital staff turnover rate has increased 30 percent in the past year and management is seen as taking little action to remedy the problem. Upper level management is also shifting roles, as a result of which her direct superior is leaving. There is speculation as to who will fill the position, but no one knows the official word. There is also a rumor that the minimum education for manager positions will become a B.S.N. degree. This would require Mary Alice to return to school to complete her degree in order to get a promotion.

In this busy area the charge nurse needs to delegate any responsibilities other than administering the floor, in order to survive. Unfortunately, Mary Alice has difficulty delegating and therefore ends up staying later or taking paperwork home. Her staff thinks she is a great clinical nurse because she frequently helps out her staff. "I don't know what my bosses think; they never tell me. I've thought about being a head nurse, but the days I am in charge are frantic."

She frequently feels guilty that she has not done enough. Mary Alice is heading for burnout because she is taking on too much work; her work life is unsatisfying and is overlapping into her personal life.

In her personal life there are several significant changes. She has bouts of loneliness since her breakup six weeks ago with her boyfriend of three years. This happened shortly after she heard that her ex-husband was remarrying. Her elderly mother and father are having some medical problems with arthritis and CHF. Her younger sister just married and she does not like the man. She notices that in coping with her feelings in response to all these difficulties, her chocolate binges have increased. She also has had more colds in the past year, requiring her to take time off from work.

Educator

Let me introduce you to another nurse on whose case this book could be based. As you read, imagine the stress she must feel.

Susan is an assistant professor in a B.S.N. program in a midwestern college. The school of nursing is expanding to include a master's program. She is already carrying 12 teaching hours and now she will carry 16 hours until new faculty can be hired. "But even if new faculty were hired, we would still be overworked," Susan said. "They would find something else for us to do, like increase the amount of research or publishing you need to do." She is also expected to serve on one university committee and one faculty committee. These increasing demands by the university have placed considerable strain on faculty–management relationships.

In order to get tenure she has to publish two articles in the next ten months. "Usually I am good at setting goals and reaching them, but I hate writing and now I am caught in 'publish or perish'." If she does not get tenure she will have to leave. With this time pressure and competition for tenure, she feels she is struggling to keep her head above water.

Her students see her as an excellent teacher—always available and well prepared for class. However, she is also known for her demanding perfectionism and can be overly critical at times. "I wonder if my students know I am just as demanding and critical of myself." Susan said, "I always thought that once you knew what your problem was you could change yourself. Unfortunately, I was wrong. Though I know I am perfectionistic and overly critical, I still can't seem to stop the behavior."

Consequently, her interpersonal relationsihps with both students and other faculty is sometimes distant. Her perfectionism carries over to her personal life, and since it is not perfect she feels upset periodically. Her children are now approaching adolescence and she is tired of their rebellious nature and the family conflicts it produces. Her husband, experiencing work pressure, is not as easygoing or attentive as he once was.

Many times she would like to escape to a quiet, secluded island. Anxiety and stomach upset are her common symptoms of stress. Recently, she was told by her family doctor that unless she changed she would become an ulcer patient within a year.

Manager

The last case study involves a middle-level nurse manager. The following is a letter from Margaret, depicting vividly what causes burnout in nurse managers.

Dear Vickie,

I have been on vacation for three weeks—the first since 1979. The world looks different when you are rested and happy! I go back to work in two days— I'm not looking forward to that.

I do not like the administrative work, especially with the work load I have in middle management. *Some* of my responsibilities follow:

- I am responsible for two buildings (24-hour basis—get called at home, work different hours, and many hours if necessary); capacity for 200 patients—10 wards.
- My subordinates include: 4 supervisors, 2 head nurses, LPNs, RNs—160 employees in all, represented by two unions.
- I am responsible for geriatric admissions, 3 wards of continued care geriatric patients, and psychiatric patients with medical problems.
- I am nursing representative on the hospital Infection Control Committee.
- I am supposed to be the liaison person between our hospital and community hospitals and visit patients who are sent here for acute illness.

- I answer grievances and attend greivance hearings when necessary.
- Three weekends in six months I am in charge of the whole hospital.
- I counsel employees that the supervisors have problems with.
- I write job descriptions, policies, procedures, recommendations, and justifications, try to schedule with insufficient staff, attend meetings, and hold meetings.
- I am responsible for the quality of nursing care given in my service, and must make sure that we meet J.C.A.H. and Medicare standards—however, I do not have any control over the amount or quality of staff in my service. I can document my heart out for months on end and finally get rid of unsatisfactory staff, but it is difficult.
- I review payroll, timekeeping, and attendance records, and building and equipment maintenance.
- I prepare the budget for my service with appropriate justifications and submit it to the nursing office, which sends it on up the line, where it is finally "scratched" in Trenton!
- Some of these responsibilities I delegate to others; I could delegate more if I had more permanent staff members and more time to train them, etc., etc., etc.,

As you can see, I am responsible for many *nonnursing* duties. I have many ideas that I don't have time to develop. I am intelligent, creative, and a good nurse. I love nursing, psychology, and psychiatry, but I am stifled and frustrated.

They tell me that I am unorganized because I cannot get all this done in eight hours a day! I have difficulty communicating upline and feel trapped, squashed, angry, and hostile at times. A "constant fail" situation creates a high degree of frustration, and I'm there! I make a sincere effort to be supportive of my staff and keep up a good front, but I frequently am not successful, I'm sure.

This situation is not a figment of my imagination, as others have noted and commented on my situation—even surveyers. I tried to get another job several years ago, but I was overqualified and overeducated—I would have taken a $7,000 cut in salary. Even though statistics prove that job satisfaction rates higher than salary, I don't think the people I talked to believe it. I have not tried since because home conditions have changed and I cannot take that much of a cut in salary.

What have I done about this? I took a course in "mind control for relaxation techniques," which helps a lot. I have also started my own business, which is growing and becoming more and more profitable, and I am starting to feel less trapped. The people I am involved with are positive, happy people and a pleasure to be around, and I feel like a different person at these times. I have just hired a bookkeeper and an accountant to free more of my time. In another year or two I will leave nursing altogether. It is a shame that nurses are forced to do this or "go crazy"—I choose, however, to enjoy the rest of my life in good mental and physical health.*

---

*Margaret did not leave nursing. She is now director of nursing for a small hospital and is enjoying nursing again.

In these histories lie many of the kernals for the ideas presented in this book. The physical, emotional, and social stressors these nurses describe are typical of those experienced by professional nurses today (Sutterly & Donnelly, 1982). I suspect that all of you reading this have experienced some of these effects from time to time. The overload of stress leads to "burnout." What do we mean by "burnout"?

DEFINITION OF THE PROBLEM:
WHAT IS BURNOUT?

Webster's New World Dictionary defines *burnout* as exhaustion from too much work or dissipation. For the purpose of this book, *burnout* is defined as physical and emotional exhaustion resulting in discernible negative responses and attitudes toward both others and oneself. First, the burnout shows in negative job attitudes; then negative attitudes toward oneself; and, finally, in a loss of feeling and concern for those one cares for. The exhaustion is due to an overload on the energy, strength, or resources of the individual. Simply put, burnout means being drained, worn out, depleted. With the demands and pressures of dealing with doctors, administrators, and other professionals while simultaneously providing quality patient care or education, is it any wonder that nurses experience burnout, or its synonomous and equally accurate term, "battle fatigue"?

Burnout is rapidly becoming the number one occupational health hazard for nursing personnel. While the signs and symptoms vary from one individual to another, there are specific and recognizable diagnostic indicators. The prognosis depends on when the individual develops an awareness of these indicators. Naturally, the earlier treatment begins, the greater the likelihood of successful extinction of symptoms. Obviously, prevention is the key. As this problem reaches epidemic proportions, it is imperative that nursing personnel and hospital administrators focus on the issues involved.

Burnout is a multidimensional problem that has replaced "reality shock" as the most talked about nursing phenomenon. The changing social and economic structure of the United States has created stressful family and career conflicts. The nursing profession itself is undergoing changes at several levels. Political infighting and competition are escalating between various factions of nurses, resulting in a lack of cooperation and support for each other personally as well as professionally.

The physical manifestations of burnout seem like a list of complaints from a text on psychosomatic medicine—fatigue, headaches, insomnia, and backaches. The body, exhausted due to overwork and high tension levels or fatiguing tasks, breaks down—with injury or disease as a result. The body is no longer able to cope and says, "I quit if you won't."

The mind quits too. As a result of the fogging effects of depression and dissociation, or the confusion associated with anxiety, the mind ceases to think clearly. Psychological problems are often manifested behaviorally, and the nurse overdoes food, alcohol, drugs, or smoking in an attempt to cope with the psychological pain. Emotional outbursts of anger or sadness and rigid, inflexible behaviors all can be seen as the mind's attempt to reduce tension and restore order.

What are the causes of these symptoms? Is burnout an inevitable problem for all nurses, or are there certain people who are more likely to break down with symptoms? What are some treatment, management, and prevention strategies available to the nurse to help her or him cope?

These questions and more will be addressed in this book for nurses on the effective management of stress and prevention of burnout. Burnout is a consequence of ineffective identification and management of stress. By identifying your stress contributors and developing strategies to deal with them, you can eradicate burnout as a problem for you.

2

Physical Strategies: Protecting Your Body

LIFESTYLE HABITS CAN CREATE ILLNESS

Chronic stress, and its consequent disease and disability is the major health problem in the United States today. We are almost free of the many infectious diseases that historically wiped out civilizations. Before the 1800s the leading causes of death were pneumonia, influenza, tuberculosis, and diarrhea/enteritis (Barnard, 1974). Chronic disease, rather than infectious diseases, became the predominant focus of the medical professions in the late 1950s. We have substituted one set of killers for another.

Actually, medical science has done little to increase the potential lifespan of the American adult. Figures quoted about the average life expectancy show an increase since the introduction of antibiotics in the 1940s. But this supposed increase is due mainly to a lower infant and childhood mortality rate. We are not really living any longer than did people 60 years ago (Kuntzleman, 1978, p. 92–94). The death rate in the United States has barely declined over the last 30 years.

The health and lifestyle habits of people today are harming individuals by leading to illness and cost business $60 billion annually in decreased productivity (Artz, 1981). The economic costs are high, yet they hardly reflect all the human costs.

Lifestyle habits such as cigarette smoking, the third martini, or that piece of chocolate-chocolate cake can no longer be seen as simply "bad habits." These habits create chronic illness that are at the top of the list as causes of death in the United States. According to the U.S. Department of Health, Education and Welfare Census, of every 100 deaths in

7

1978, 38 were due to heart disease, 21 to cancer, 9 to stroke, and 6 to accidents; 48 percent of accidental deaths were due to motor vehicles (Russell, 1980).

Long-term abuse takes a variety of forms. For some nurses it is the lack of exercise or an inadequate diet that takes a toll on the body's functioning. The body shows this abuse with flabby muscles, inflexibility, and midriff bulge.

Other nurses have lifestyle habits that include the use of drugs that stimulate the body, such as caffeine or "pep" pills. On the "down" side are sleeping pills and assorted pain and tranquilizing drugs to slow the mind and body, thus dulling stress. This abuse of the body will eventually show in signs, then symptoms, and then illness if the habits are not changed.

Each day as a nurse you have some contact with the effects of disease and poor health habits. Perhaps you also see the effects in your own family. You are not immune. It is important that you find better ways to manage stress. The purpose of this chapter is to convince you to begin to take seriously the statement "with everything we do to our bodies and minds, we are either promoting health or fostering illness."

You will come to understand this statement first by realizing how stress affects your body. Your body's response to threat is based upon a self-protective "fight or flight" response. All perceived threats stimulate this biological response. Most threats to your well-being today are not physical threats, but are threats to your ego. Someone criticizing you for a mistake can set in motion the same mechanism as the San Francisco earth trembling beneath your feet. Unfortunately, most people don't know they are also triggering this mechanism with dysfunctional habits such as the consumption of sugar, caffeine, pep pills, and nicotine.

You then have the opportunity to assess the types of signs and symptoms you are most vulnerable to. Abuse to your body can lead to gastrointestinal problems, which could, with long-term abuse, develop into ulcers or colitis. Taking a look at your "family illness tree" (see Fig. 2-2) will help you identify some of your vulnerable areas. Some authors refer to these as the "weak links" of the body. Knowing your biological weak links is important in determining your prevention strategies. The signs and symptoms checklist (see Table 2-2) will raise your level of awareness of your body's natural warning system.

After you have considered the role of heredity, the most important consideration is lifestyle habits and environmental conditions. These factors are very important in managing stress, for to some degree they are controllable. Lifestyle factors, such as being a nonexerciser and overworking affect the quality of your life and your stress level. Add environmental conditions such as a high-stress job in a high-crime area, and you are fostering a significant stress level.

Finally, physical habits that can be developed to relieve stress on your body and your mind are surveyed. The basic premise is that what relaxes your mind relaxes your muscles. Fortunately, it is also true that what relaxes your muscles can relax your mind. This gives you a choice of many methods.

Some methods involve focusing your mind for relaxation and other methods work directly on relaxing your muscles. A key to relieving tension that affects all body parts is to reduce all behavior that places unnecessary wear and tear on the body. A second key is to engage in behavior—such as relaxation and physical exercise—that allows your body to revitalize its internal healing processes. In this chapter we focus on the second key.

HOW THE BODY HANDLES STRESS

Consider the following scenario: You go to check a postoperative patient's dressing and find him in a pool of blood. He is difficult to arouse and his color is pale. Instantly, your heart pounds, your body tenses, and 1000 alternatives race through your mind. Your blood pressure leaps; stored sugar is released into your blood stream. Then, just as you are about to yell for help, you wake up and realize you were dreaming. Within minutes you return to normal, left with nothing more than the shakiness of an adrenalin hangover.

This incident is perceived and interpreted by your brain cortex to be a stressor. The cortex triggers the hypothalmus, and the hypothalmus is in charge of triggering the anterior and posterior pituitary. The anterior pituitary secretes the hormone adrenocorticotropin (ACTH), which makes the adrenal glands secrete several hormones, providing strength to do battle or run away. As you will see, this is the beginning of a triggering process set up by the body.

The thyroid gland, pancreas, and adrenals are also affected by the release of hormones; the important fact to realize is that once the message is sent to begin the triggering process, the entire body is affected. This process is depicted in Figure 2-1. Follow the process through your body once and perhaps you can begin to understand the importance of doing something about your stress level.

The following review of the anatomy and physiology involved in the processes shown in Figure 2-1 will help you understand the significance of the stress response to your physical health; the physiology of this response affects all systems of the body. This discussion is focused on the endocrine and cardiovascular systems.

The hypothalamus controls the autonomic nervous system functions,

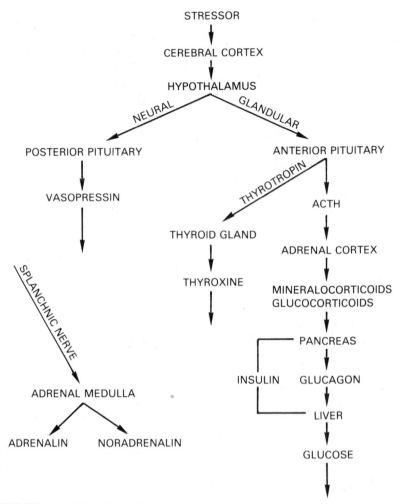

FIGURE 2-1.   How the body reacts to stress.

coordinating circulation, digestion, and other processes not normally under conscious control. As it receives the fight or flight message from the cortex, it immediately signals the master gland, the pituitary, to begin its work. Thus the hypothalamus can be seen as the part of the brain responsible for the triggering of the body's hormonal and neural responses to stress.

The pituitary gland has two lobes. The posterior lobe is mostly neural tissue, and when stimulated it releases the hormone vasopressin. The contraction of the arteries, and therefore the raising of the blood pressure, is due to vasopressin.

The anterior pituitary gland is mostly glandular in nature and is responsible for six of the major hormones. Only two of these are directly involved in the stress response: ACTH is the first, and thyrotropin is the second. The former triggers the adrenal cortex and the latter stimulates the thyroid gland.

The stimulated thyroid gland secretes thyroxine, the chief thyroid hormone. Thyroxine raises the metabolic rate to prepare the body to take action in response to the stressor. The heart rate increases and breathing becomes deep and rapid.

ACTH triggers the adrenal cortex to produce proinflammatory and anti-inflammatory corticoids. There are over 30 of these corticoids, but they break down into two groups—mineralocorticoids and glucocorticoids. The mineralocorticoids, by their influence on the kidney, promote inflammation.

Glucocorticoids are anti-inflammatory in action; they are the corticoids primarily affected by ACTH. Cholesterol is reduced by ACTH action. Glucocorticoids raise the sugar level of the body by stimulating the pancrease to produce glucagon.

Glucagon raises the sugar level by stimulating the liver to release stored sugar. Insulin also is released by the pancreas and is the antagonist to glucagon. Insulin moves the sugar out of the blood into the cells, thus lowering the blood sugar levels. In the stress response two hormones are working to raise the sugar level—glucocorticoids and adrenalin—and insulin alone is secreted to lower the sugar levels. Perhaps this helps explain why insulin-producing cells begin to break down through overwork, thus producing diabetes.

The adrenal medulla is the other section of the adrenal gland and is primarily nervous tissue. The splanchnic nerve triggers the medulla to secrete adrenalin and noradrenalin. Both of these hormones equip you for emergency action by acting mainly on the cardiovascular and metabolic systems. This action was described eariler.

The effects of stress upon the body involve all major glands and organs. The body is literally bathed in hormones, and organs are triggered to perform through their chemical reactions. As you can imagine, chronic triggering of this mechanism can wear out the machine parts. The part you wear out depends upon several factors.

HEREDITY AND FAMILY ATTITUDE

Figure 2-2 suggests a convenient method for assessing potentially vulnerable health areas. Once the family illness tree has been completely filled out, you should look carefully for any repeat of illnesses. There is

```
FATHER'S FAMILY                          MOTHER'S FAMILY

Grandmother      Grandfather             Grandmother      Grandfather
_____      _____             _____      _____
_____      _____             _____      _____
_____      _____             _____      _____

Your Father                              Your Mother
_____                   _____
_____                   _____
_____                   _____

Aunt(s)          Uncle(s)                Aunt(s)          Uncle(s)
_____      _____             _____      _____
_____      _____             _____      _____
_____      _____             _____      _____


Your Brother(s)                          Your Sister(s)
_____                _____
_____                _____
_____                _____

                 You
                 _____
                 _____
                 _____
```

Physical	Psychological
Heart and artery disease	Depression
Hypertension	Anxiety neurosis
Kidney disease	Schizophrenia
Diabetes	Manic-depressive illness
Hypoglycemia	Paranoia
Liver disease	
Gallbladder disease	*Behavioral*
Migraine headaches	Alcoholism
Arthritis	Drug addiction
Lung disease	(includes cigarettes,
Cancer	caffeine, and sugar)
	Accidents

FIGURE 2-2. Family illness tree. This tree can aid in the assessment of potentially vulnerable health areas. Under each family member would be listed any chronic problems he or she had; cause of death would also be listed. Under the tree itself is a list to choose from.

research evidence that certain illnesses run in families. If you notice a pattern in your family tree, certain chapters of this book may be particularly relevant. For instance, if heart disease appears in several places, then this chapter will be of special interest: exercise and relaxation are known treatment and prevention strategies for heart disease.

Look at your family tree in terms of illnesses listed at the time of death. Your father may have died of cancer, but had paralysis or loss of speech from a stroke for years beforehand. What caused the stroke? An embolism from artery disease or an embolism from uncorrected mitral stenosis? The second one is a correctable problem left unattended.

Another important contribution from your family is their attitude toward health and illness. If you come from a family that believes "all of us Salvios are destined to die of heart attacks" or "all Lutzes get diabetes later in life" you have been conditioned to believe you will too. "Conditioned to believe" is different than "destined to die." Consider the genetic predisposition, but do not give up responsibility for your lifestyle habits with an attitude of "destined to."

One final word about one of the major causes of death in the United States that is being seen as strongly psychosocially connected—cancer. LeShan (1959) in reviewing the literature from 1902 to 1957, found life stresses and psychiatric illnesses associated with cancer. Depression, hopelessness, and grief emerged as frequently cited precursors to cancer. Hurst and associates (1976), in their review, linked depression and anxiety with the subsequent development of malignant tumors. Cancer, a physical disease, seems to occur more frequently in people with the tendency to respond to stress with decreased energy and emotional withdrawal (Hagnell, 1966; Thomas & Greenstreet, 1973). Cancer, then, like the many other diseases listed previously, is connected with how you deal with stress.

PHYSICAL SIGNS AND SYMPTOMS OF STRESS

Continue your physical assessment by reviewing what, if any, signs and symptoms you presently have that are related to stress. Dealing with these signs and symptoms could prevent later consequences of disease. Table 2-1 itemizes the physical signs and symptoms of stress. List those that you have had in the past 6 months. Make another list of the ones that are of most concern for you today. Make up a third list of those items that are or could become a chronic problem for you. These are the ones to keep especially in mind when you are thinking about your health.

These are signs and symptoms of various physical and psychological diseases. The quality and the intensity of these symptoms may vary, but

Table 2-1
PHYSICAL SIGNS AND SYMPTOMS OF STRESS

Increased heart rate
Elevated blood pressure
Tightness of chest
Breathing difficulty
Headaches, migraine
Fatigue, exhaustion
Insomnia
Gastrointestinal problems: nausea, diarrhea, vomiting, intestinal disturbances, ulcers, colitis, stomach aches
Restlessness, hyperactivity
Vague somatic complaints, feeling rundown, minor ailments, psychosomatic complaints
Backaches
Frequent or prolonged colds or flu
Bruxism, clenching
Urinary frequency
Weight gain or weight loss of more than 10 pounds

---

they all need to be considered in assessing your physical health. Some are warnings that your body is not functioning normally. Especially note the ones you have listed that were absent two years ago. Finally, note the ones that are increasing. List your major concerns.

Hans Seyle, the founding father of stress research, explains the process of body breakdown with the theory called general adaptation syndrome (Selye, 1974). Symptoms of stress can occur at any of the three stages in this syndrome: alarm, resistance, and exhaustion. These three stages form the biological stress syndrome. The animal experiments conducted by Seyle (1976) showed that the body has a finite amount of adaptation energy to deal with stress. Once we have made a withdrawal from our adaptation energy account, there seems to be no way to make a replacement deposit.

In the initial, alarm stage, the body responds to the stressors by mobilizing its defenses to deal with the threat. The stage of resistance begins as the body fights back. Just as the boxer in the ring who is having a tough fight begins to wear down, so does the body. In the stage of exhaustion the body no longer can "stand up and fight." As a nurse you see these stages of response in your patients as they cope with the stress of illness.

People spend varying amounts of time in each of these stages. At present there is no conclusive proof that we can add years to our life by better handling of these stress stages. However, the quality of life can improve. Your signs and symptoms are warning lights bidding you to pay attention to your body. Early recognition and treatment of these warnings will improve the quality of your life.

Psychomatic illness is the most frequently used diagnosis: 80 percent of the people who see general practice doctors are said to have a psychosomatic illness. Nicely put, this means the patient has a disease with a psychological connection. Too often, this person is sloughed off as "a head job" and is treated with tranquilizers or told to relax. Unfortunately, most people who are told to relax need help in learning how to do it.

This idea that the state of the mind affects the body is well accepted in the medical community. What is less understood is the role of these psychosocial factors in preserving health. Psychosocial factors play a role in all illnesses.

Valliant (1979) did a 40-year study on 95 healthy young men and found that how they mastered stress, that is, their adaptation mode, was more significant than the quality and quantity of their stress. He found that psychological factors played a role in determining whether they remained physically healthy. Psychological defense mechanisms allow the individual to reclaim comfort or prevent the discomfort of uncontrollable and sudden changes. Valliant describes our defense mechanisms as analogous to the white blood cells battling diseases on a physical level.

The four classes of defenses are divided into three categories that lead to unhealthy behavior and one that encompasses the mature, desirable mechanisms. The first three classes lead to psychotic and neurotic behaviors, as well as personality disorders. The mature mechanisms include humor, altruism, sublimation, and suppression. The men who remained in excellent health showed predominantly these mature defenses. Of the healthy men 80 percent exhibited these mechanisms. The men with the other defense mechanisms were likely to show signs of illness or disability.

The reasons for this finding are not clear at present. Perhaps the mature defenses bind these people to other people and thereby provide individuals with the support that reduces stress. These defenses are learnable and perhaps need to be part of the stress reduction curriculum.

Your body can begin to break down when it becomes unbalanced by perceived threats to your well-being. Many of the threats are threats to your ego rather than physical threats. Often, because the threat is not visible, individuals do not associate their stress level, their physical well-being, and their life changes as being connected. The threat of criticism can trigger the body into the same biological processes as a visible bear. You need to recognize these threats and begin to take constructive action to remedy the triggering process.

Table 2-2
ENVIRONMENTAL CONDITIONS AND LIFESTYLE
HABITS RELATED TO STRESS

Environmental conditions	Lifestyle
High level of pollution	Smoker
Live/work with smokers	Drinker
High-stress job	Overeater
In management position without skills	Little/no physical exercise
	Overwork
Hazardous job	Hectic life
Live/work in high-crime area	Use drugs
Need to be in one position for extended periods of time	Drink coffee/tea
	High fat/sugar diet
Repeated x-ray exposure	Type A personality
Exposure to radioactive drugs	Ingest chemical-laden foods
Exposure to toxic chemical irritants	Eat processed and refined foods
	Poor health habits (checkups less than twice a year for dentist, less than 6 months–1 year for gynecologist)

ENVIRONMENTAL CONDITIONS AND LIFESTYLE FACTORS

The illness you are likely to develop is related to your environment and your lifestyle as well as your psychological state. Working in an asbestos plant or a coal mine and getting asbestosis or black lung is strong evidence for environmental factors creating diseases.

Take a minute to assess yourself by listing those factors in Table 2-2 that apply to you. If you find you have an environmental condition and a lifestyle habit that relate to each other, please begin to consider some changes in your life. Having combinations of these factors increases your chances of illness. For instance, if an individual has a history of heart disease and also lifestyle factors such as smoking, overeating, lack of physical exercise, and a Type A personality, then these add up to five known factors contributing to the development of heart disease. For years health educators have tried to get people to take these as serious factors. Practicing positive health habits is as important as teaching them.

No matter how much you choose to deny the importance of poor health habits by thinking "it won't happen to me," in reality their effect on your genetic predisposition needs to be taken seriously. Begin to take seriously what you learned in the last self-assessment. You cannot take control of your genes, but you can take control of your lifestyle and some environmental factors.

We often forget that environmental conditions are a factor in creating illness. What you breathe or ingest into your body affects your body's ability to function normally—to maintain its homeostatic balance. If you live in a high-crime area and work in a high-stress job, your environmental conditions support continuous high stress levels. Your body breaks down when it can no longer cope with the internal tension. Where you work and live plays a role in maintaining your health.

Numerous studies (Gentry, Foster, & Froehling, 1972; Ivancevich & Matteson, 1980; Oskins, 1979) point to the high levels of work stress in ICU and non-ICU settings. Some aspects of this environmental stress can be changed. Gentry et al. (1972) suggest some causes of work stress based on their study results: "The psychologic response evidenced on the various tests appeared to be associated with situational stress including an overwhelming workload, too much responsibility, poor communication between nurses and physicians, limited work space, and too little continuing education" (p. 796). Sound familiar? Work as an environmental stress factor needs close consideration.

If you are a public health nurse in North Philadelphia or New York City, you work in hazardous job conditions. No matter now much you choose to deny it, your environmental work conditions are stressful. Also beware if smoking is checked in the lifestyle column of your self-assessment (Table 2-2)—96 percent of the people with lung cancer smoked.

METHODS OF STRESS REDUCTION

There are two keys to managing your health in order to treat and prevent physical burnout. The first is to have relaxation times for healing and rejuvenation, and the second is to train your body to withstand stress through exercise. Part of the training in relaxation involves direct relaxation of muscles and other techniques that involve calming the mind, and thereby relaxing the body.

The treatments are logical when you understand how stress affects your body. As you followed the description of the process in the second section, the effects upon the entire body became obvious. The signs and symptoms you checked in Table 2-1 are your warnings that your body is not handling stress effectively. Unfortunately, many people do not perceive their history, environmental conditions, and lifestyle factors as causal in their level of stress. In the preceding section, the relationship among all these factors was emphasized. In this section alternative ways of coping with the inevitable stress of nursing are offered.

Physical burnout is caused by the body's coping responses overworking to the point where a part of the system breaks down. The machine part stops working effectively or stops completely. Remember your vulnerable system and your vulnerable body part from the previous exercises. In this section we focus on how you can best treat the effects of the problem and also prevent further breakdown.

Muscle Relaxation and Tension Release

Muscle relaxation and changing lifestyle habits are the two main techniques to prevent and treat physical burnout. Muscle relaxation techniques discussed here are not all inclusive; they are the main ones I have seen used with some degree of success and, at times, cure. Since physical exercise involves muscle relaxation, flexibility, and strengthening, it is included in this chapter; other lifestyle habit changes are discussed in other chapters.

The premises upon which treatment and prevention are based include the following:

- Muscles relax when tension is released.
- Focusing your mind on the tense muscles or on a relaxing image relaxes muscles.
- Activity is a way to relax muscles.
- Activity can be seen as a means of energy discharge or as an attention diversion.

You can relax muscles by concentrating on something relaxing (diversion) or by focusing directly on the muscle with a "relax" message. Any experience that does either will decrease your internal tension. Regular practice of any of the following relaxation methods will help decrease your muscle tension level and decrease your response to stressors in general. Muscles can be taught to relax and to be relaxed even under stressful conditions.

Biofeedback is a muscle relaxation technique taught through the use of a machine. By monitoring your muscle in your forehead by means of an electromyogram (EMG) or testing your galvanic skin response (GSR) in your index finger, the machine indicates to you your state of relaxation. By observing a flashing red light turning yellow and then green, a tone decreasing in magnitude, you can identify a decrease in your body tension.

During biofeedback sessions you may also practice relaxing your muscles by focusing on a relaxing image (Brown, 1974). Audiotapes of the sound of waves and visual imagery are often used to facilitate creating relaxing images. After a period of practice you will have learned to recognize your various levels of muscle tension and relaxation, and if you consistently continue to practice after the biofeedback sessions cease, you will continue to achieve muscle relaxation. I have seen this method work very effectively for migraine and tension headache sufferers.*

It has been established that a combination of EMG feedback training and home practice in relaxation is very effective in the treatment of tension headaches. Several studies have shown headaches eliminated or markedly reduced (Adler & Adler, 1976; Budzynski, Sloyva, & Adler, 1970; Wiekramaskekera, 1972). Biofeedback, like any method to reduce tension, must be practiced for the effects to be continuous.

Autogenic training is often used in conjunction with biofeedback. This deep-relaxation technique was developed by the German psychiatrist Johannes H. Schutz in 1932. Persons who, for whatever reason, are not interested in meditative techniques might consider autogenic training. The idea behind the training is that brief sessions of concentration produce a state of relaxation. Information on this technique is available in several publications (Davis, Eshelman, & McKay, 1980; Pelletier, 1977; Rosa, 1973; Shealy, 1977).

Proponents of autogenic training have devised six exercises for the regulation of circulation, respiration, and neuromuscular activity. The first component is a series of self-suggestion relaxation phrases. The second group of exercises consists of single-focus mental concentration, similar to meditation. The four types of exercises are described in the books cited above. The benefits of continued use have allowed individuals to dispense with the use of medications for relaxation and pain relief.

Hypnosis and self-hypnosis have been practiced for hundreds of years in childbirth and as forms of anesthesia. Self-hypnosis is a tool that can be used to reduce stress and to achieve a state of relaxation that renders the individual receptive to autosuggestion for dealing with a problem. Sleep is not needed for hypnosis; instead a state is brought about that allows the subconscious mind to be communicated with. These fascinating techniques of hypnosis and self-hypnosis are discussed and taught in a number of books (Davis, et al., 1980; Haley, 1967; LeCron, 1970; Morris, 1974).

Massage is a method of muscle relaxation (Downing, 1972). Massage, whether superficial or deep, creates a relax message from the outside to the inside. The muscles send the message to the brain via the nerve pathways, creating a gradual light sensation as the stress level abates. There are many legitimate masseurs and massage therapists.

---

*If you are interested in learning these techniques ask your doctor for a referral or send a stamped, self-addressed envelope to the Biofeedback Society of America, 4301 Owens Street, Wheat Ridge, CO 80033.

Check at your health club or holistic health center for the name of a local person. Health food stores and your local humanistic psychologists would probably also know of a few.

If you never have had a massage, do treat yourself to an experience that could be addictive. In fact, I believe it is the one way some men have legitimized in their heads a way to get touched nurturingly. Medicine that feels this good could make you a believer in the merits of holistic health.

Reflexology is a concentrated massage of the soles of the feet (Bergson & Tuchack, 1974). It works on the principles of acupressure, using the pressure points in the soles of the feet. Pains in organs and muscles far removed from the area are affected by stimulation of these nerve endings because these points are related to meridians, or energy channels, that crisscross the body.

Kinesiology, the scientific study of movement, applies the organizing principles of anatomy, physiology, and physics to the mechanisms of movement. It includes many modalities, such as rolfing and bioenergetics. These modalities, like reflexology, are viewed skeptically by many in the medical profession. Health practitioners in holistic health and wellness see them all as possible treatment choices for the countering of the effects of prolonged, chronic stress.

Rolfing is a deep fascial massage. It is used not for relaxing, but for getting rid of long-term, conditioned tension in muscles due to past psychological or physical trauma. The theory states that the release of the fascia creates a relaxation in the tension of muscles. There is a systematic procedure with some focusing on the individual's problem areas (Rolf, 1977).*

Bioenergetics therapy, like rolfing, focuses on the muscular tensions of the body, a condition caused by suppression of feelings. Through the use of bioenergetic exercises, these tensions can be dissolved, thus enabling the individual to be emotionally and physically free of tension (Lowen, 1976).†

Progressive Relaxation and Visual Imagery

Creating relaxing images in your mind, combined with a progressive muscle relaxation exercise, will effectively put you in an alpha state (Jacobson, 1974). In the following exercises you focus on your various body parts, from the tips of your toes to the top of your head. This allows your muscles to relax as your mind becomes focused. After your muscles relax,

---

*Additional articles are available through the Rolf Institute, P.O. Box 1868, Boulder, CO 80306.

†For more information on this body–mind approach contact Dr. Alexander Lowen, Institute of Bioenergetic Analysis, 144 E. 36th Street, New York, NY 10016.

you create a calm, tranquil scene in your mind through the process of visualization.

Visualization simply means creating an image or a picture in your mind's eye (Donovan, 1981). You visualize a place that offers you a sense of calmness and serenity. It is probably a place you have been before and usually is an outdoor scene. Put no people in your scene.

In order to use the following relaxation exercises and the calm scene you will need to read these instructions several times and then go practice. You also could make your own relaxation tape from the directions. Your relaxation response needs to be triggered more often, so take 15 minutes now and complete this exercise. Please read the directions first.

This relaxation exercise involves focusing your attention on your body parts. Begin by taking in three deep breaths. Breathe in relaxation and exhale stress. Turn your attention now to focusing on your left foot. I suggest you use the following phrasing:

Focus on the sole of your left foot. Focus on the sole of your left foot. Focus on the sole of your left foot. Now, focus on the top of your left foot. Focus on the top of your left foot. Focus on the top of your left foot.

Continue this, repeating the focusing on the body parts. Go up one leg and then the other focusing on the shin, calf, knee, thigh, and hip. Next do the torso (belly, chest, back). Then do one arm (palm, wrist, forearm, elbow, upper arm, shoulder), go across the shoulders, including the neck, and down the other arm. Finally, do your head by including the forehead, eyes, nose, cheeks, lips, and chin. This whole process takes 9–12 minutes.

Now that you are relaxed you can begin your visualization of the calm scene. Imagine before you a huge white screen. On this screen, paint a scene that makes you feel calm. It may be a scene of the ocean, a lake, a stream. A forest scene or a snow scene may come to your mind. As several scenes may compete for your attention, pick one that best supports you relaxing. Put no people in the scene, only you and your surroundings. Visualize the blue of the sky and water, the white of the clouds or snow. Make the sun a brilliant yellow and the grass a true green. Whatever colors you use, make them clear, like a sharp picture.

As you are visualizing your scene, incorporate into the scene the sounds associated with the image. These sounds may be of birds, rain on a roof, lapping of waves, leaves rustling, or other sounds of Mother Nature. Whatever the sounds, focus the sounds as you see your scene.

As you look and hear your scene, incorporate any smell that you would connect with the scene. It may be the smell of flowers, of evergreens, or the briny smell of the ocean. A fire burning fall leaves may cast its scent, or you may smell freshly cut grass.

Now that you see the scene, hear its sounds, and smell its smell, do one final thing. Feel the scene by feeling the sun or the breeze on your skin. Reach down and feel the grass, sand, or water. Feel what is around you so that you are firmly planted in the scene.

This experience can be recreated to trigger your relaxation response. Using this method once or twice a day will create relaxation effects that last far beyond these 15 minutes. Use this exercise to relax your body and calm your mind. Allow time to return to a level of alertness. Do not rush back into high gear; it jolts your senses too much.

Meditation and Breathing

Meditation can have the same effect on your body as this relaxation exercise. Your mind also becomes calm because you are focusing on only one thing. There are two differences that have been repeatedly noted after experiencing both relaxation exercises and meditation. The first benefit is that your level of concentration improves. You begin to realize that your memory seems to be getting better. What has actually occurred is that you have been concentrating more on what is going on and therefore miss less. The second benefit is in the spiritual realm of exploration. You begin to realize how we are all alike beneath our various customs and roles. You feel like being nicer to people and are more interested in your fellow human beings. The benefit to you is that you feel good about yourself because you feel this way toward other people.

Without sounding like a medicine show man selling a cure for what ails you, I want to emphasize that meditation has profoundly affected many people's lives. Both healthy people and people with illnesses such as hypertension (Benson, Rosner, Marzetta, & Klemchuk, 1974) and drug addiction (Benson, 1967) have shown significant improvement.

Meditation needs to be practiced for at least 20 minutes daily. This consistent practice allows you to become good at concentrating, and by concentrating on yourself, you learn a great deal about yourself. Your goal is to concentrate on your breathing. The power of breathing as part of meditation has been illustrated by Zen monks in Japan who are able to reduce their oxygen consumption by as much as 20 percent.

Your pattern of breathing changes as you breath deeper and more completely. Most of the time we are breathing very shallowly. In fact, the higher the stress, the less regular and deep your breathing (Spreads, 1978). You focus all your attention on your breathing in meditation.

The pattern to follow is to breathe into your center, which is your heart, and then exhale completely. When other thoughts pass in your mind, just return your thoughts to your breathing (as soon as you recognize you have wandered away). Focus on your in-breath and your out-breath in meditation, and your mind will begin to be clearer when you are not meditating.

If you are interested in learning more, there are a number of meditation centers and classes all over the United States. Weekend or six-week courses are the most common ways to learn; there are also a number of books on meditation (LeShan, 1974; Muktananda, 1981; Naranjo & Ornstein, 1971).

Physical Fitness

Activity relaxes muscles through the discharge of tension build-up. When you experience a threatening stimulus, an emergency fight or flight reaction is immediately elicited and your muscles tighten for action. Excitation of your sympathetic nervous system results in adrenalin secretion and subsequent blood pressure and heart rate elevation, as well as other body arousal physiological changes. This physiological excitation requires discharge. Animals fight or flee and thereby discharge energy through motor activity.

For humans, norms and rules often preclude the fight or flight response. Clubbing your supervisor or your "favorite surgeon" is not an accepted mode of behavior in our civilized society. Swallowing the feelings of anger and frustration are acceptable; however, swallowing feelings whole is very bad for your body. You need instead to dissipate the energy of arousal through activity. As Gal and Lazarus (1975, p. 17) point out, "Even non-relevant activity under stress has stress-reducing capabilities in that it allows for reasonably rapid dissipation of body arousal." In other words, the activity chosen does not have to relate to the perceived threat. Physical fitness plays a role in reducing the level of catecholamines in your system, which increases with stress.

"*Physical fitness* is the ability to carry out daily tasks with vigor and alertness, without undue fatigue, and have ample energy to engage in leisure time pursuits and to meet the above average physical stresses encountered in emergency situations." (Clarke, 1979). (Definition adopted by President's Council on Physical Fitness and the American Academy of Physical Education). The components of physical fitness are interrelated, with each contributing an essential element to the human being; muscular strength, muscular endurance, and circulatory–respiratory endurance are overt manifestations of physical fitness.

There are basically three types of fitness: muscular, skeletal, and cardiovascular. Muscular fitness is developed by toning and strengthening your muscles through exercises. Calisthentics classes, Nautilus machines, and health spa programs deal mainly in the business of firming your muscles. Cavemen got plenty of muscle exercise in running, climbing, and building. You, as a nurse, probably do not exercise your muscles sufficiently for tone or strength. The one exception may be ICU nurses. As I remember my four years in the ICU, I did a lot of lifting, bending, pushing, and pulling of heavy weights!

Skeletal exercises improve the body's flexibility through simple

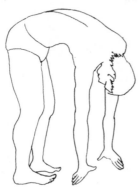

1

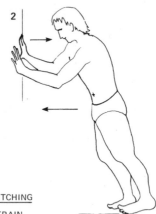

2

RULES OF STRETCHING

- NO PAIN, NO STRAIN
- NO BOUNCING WHEN STRETCHING
- RELAX AND ENJOY

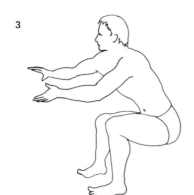

3

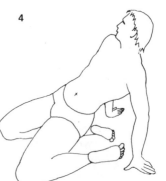

4

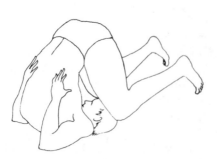

5

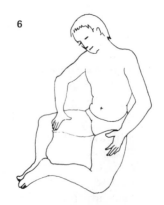

6

stretching. Six flexibility exercises are depicted in Figure 2-3. Begin these exercises with the thought of *gradually* increasing your flexibility. Many of you may require months of practice to be able to attain these positions comfortably. Flexibility exercises have proven to be very useful in preventing and treating neck and back tension and strain.

The third type of fitness is cardiopulmonary, that is, the fitness of your heart and blood vessels and your respiratory system. This can be developed by the aerobic exercises that were popularized by Cooper (1970). Running, jogging, fast-paced walking, swimming, bicycling all fall in this category.

This type of fitness is good not only for your body—surveys have shown that one of the main benefits of active participation in sports is a feeling of well-being. In a 1978 national survey* of 17,000 Americans conducted over two years, women outpaced men in taking up sports; 73 percent of the women participating started running during those two years. The survey categorized responses into four activity groups: high, moderate, low, and nonactive. Almost all participants in the active groups (80 percent) reported feeling better in general. Those in the highly active group said they had a better self-image, looked better, were more able to cope, and were more assertive and creative than before exercising. An onsite running program for Stanford University Hospital, California, nurses revealed that "a physical fitness program which focuses on running can contribute to stress reduction and well-being in nurses" (Zindler-Wernet & Bailey, 1980, p. 37).

If you feel averse to exercising, walking may be a way for you to

---

*Survey conducted for Perrier Bottled Water Co. by Louis Harris & Associates, 1978.

FIGURE 2-3. Stretching exercises for improving skeletal fitness. (1) Bend over and touch toes, gradually stretching more and more until you can place your hands flat on the floor. Reach as far as you can *without feeling pain*. Your body, through the practice of stretching, will allow you to touch your toes, and eventually the floor. (2) Lean against a wall with your arms extended, then flex your arms and you will feel the stretch up the back of your legs. This exercise stretches the muscle groups of your upper leg, calf, and Achilles tendon. (3) Squat with your heels on the floor and arms extended. You will feel the stretching in the back of your legs. (4) Lean back over flexed legs. This exercise stretches the muscles in the front of your legs. (5) Roll your legs over your head so that your knees touch the floor. *Do not push* this roll-over, otherwise you could injure lower back muscles. This exercise stretches lower back muscles—very important for nurses' backs. (6) Place your heels together and press down on your knees with your hands to stretch the thigh muscles. [Adapted from Anderson, R. The perfect pre-run stretching routine. *Runner's World,* 1978, *13,* 57–61.]

Table 2-3
WHAT'S IN WALKING FOR YOU?

Question: Are the following statements true or false?

Walking can be as efficient an aerobic exercise as jogging or running.
The distance you walk can be more important than the speed.
Walking is a form of endurance training.
If you walk briskly 20 minutes a day more than you usually do, you will lose one
    pound in 36 days, and ten pounds in a year.
If you walk one hour a day more than you usually do, in a year you will lose 30
    pounds.
You can ease anxiety by walking.
Walking is a partial defense against heavy smoking.
Menstrual discomforts are relieved by walking.
If you have just had an operation, walking usually hastens your convalescence.
Vigorous walking is a natural laxative.
Walking helps you to sleep.
Bones exercised by walking are less likely to break.
The most practical lifelong exercise is walking.
Daily walking is an "antiage antibiotic."
Walking helps guard postmenopausal women against heart attacks.
Walking is one of the greatest freedoms and pleasures of life.

Reprinted from Rudner, R. Walking, the no. 1 exercise for head, heart, and body. *Self,*
1979, *4,* 74. With permission.
Answers: All of the above statements are true.

begin a physical fitness program. Join the other 90 million Americans and
get some form of exercise. For 34 million the good old-fashioned walk is
that main exercise. Take the quiz presented in Table 2-3 and see how
informed you are about the benefits of this exercise.

A 20-minute walk at a comfortable pace is the usual recommendation. This is your first goal, not your starting point if you have been doing
little or no exercise. Increase your time and pace gradually. The condi-
tioning effects of walking improve dramatically at speeds faster than three
miles an hour that are sustained for at least 20 minutes. The President's
Council on Physical Fitness recommends an eventual goal of three miles
in 45 minutes and a minimum of three walks every week.*

---

*Three valuable resources are available to you if you choose walking for your exercise
program. The *Complete Book of Walking* by Knutzleman (1982) offers valuable suggestions.
Walking for Exercise and Pleasure, a booklet by the President's Council on Physical Fitness
and Sports, is available free by writing to 400 Sixth Street, S.W., Suite 3030, Washington,
D.C. 20201. Finally, a newsletter, walking tour guidebooks, and other services are available
to fee-paying members of the Walking Association, 4113 Lee Highway, Arlington, VA
22207.

Table 2-4
TRAINING ZONE CALCULATION

1. To find your maximum heart rate, subtract your age from 220:
   $$220 - 35 = 185$$
2. To find your appropriate pulse range, multiply 70 percent and 85 percent by your maximum heart rate (to be in your training zone you need to be functioning at 70–85 percent of your maximum heart rate):
   $$.70 \times 185 = 130$$
   $$.85 \times 185 = 157$$
3. If you stood still for one minute to feel for this pulse rate, your pulse would drop and you would fail to get an accurate measure, therefore instead you take it for ten seconds. To find the appropriate pulse rate for ten seconds, you divide your maximum pulse rate and minimum pulse rate by 6:
   $$130/6 = 22$$
   $$147/6 = 26$$

Adapted from American Heart Association. *Standards for supervised cardiovascular excercise maintenance programs.* Dallas, TX, 1980.

One of the key points in exercising, whether it is walking or any other form, is that in order for it to make a difference you need to do it consistently three or four times a week, for 15–30 minutes, in your training zone. These are the three ingredients for the FIT formula—the frequency, intensity, and time. This will produce a training effect in 12–16 weeks. The *training zone* is the range between the minimum and maximum number of heartbeats per minute that will result in the training effect for a healthy person without working so hard as to produce stress or working so little as to produce results only very slowly.

In order to calculate your training zone, follow the American Heart Association (1980) standards and formula presented above. To follow this formula simply substitute the correct figures for you. The age of 35 is used as an example. If you are 35 years old and in good health, you would need to exercise three or four times a week for 15–30 minutes with a pulse rate equivalent to 22–26 beats for a ten second period to maintain cardiopulmonary fitness. This formula is designed for a healthy person. If you have heart disease or other diseases affecting your general health, this formula will need to be altered. If you are 15 percent over your normal weight, this rate would also need to be lowered. Check with your doctor before beginning an exercise program.

Do not do exercise in order to lose weight. A physical fitness program begun for a purpose other than its own sake often ends up nowhere. Exercise needs to be done for its own sake: 40–60 percent of those who begin an exercise program quit within the first six months; they end up injured or discouraged because they expected too much too fast and did not develop their program gradually. You need 12–16 weeks to habituate yourself to an exercise program. Find an exercise you enjoy and do it consistently, and eventually you will see the differences.

Diversion

Activities unrelated to the cause of stress can have stress-reducing effects. By distracting or diverting your attention from the stress cues, you can decrease your tension level. Studies have shown repeatedly that an individual's responses are immediately reduced or eliminated when attention is diverted. Focusing your attention on something other than the threatening situation allows you to relax in body and mind.

Activity diversions can be as active as gardening or as quiet as needlepoint. Doing pottery or weaving, volunteering at the local Sierria Club or Population Zero—such activities support your creativity or contribute to your world. Using these activities to relax is a positive use of diversion.

PREVENTION TACTICS

Wellness Philosophy

The wellness philosophy views health as more than the absence of disease. You are either promoting health or promoting disease by the way you run your life. If you choose to skip lunch because you are just too busy and instead have a cigarette break, then you must recognize that you have chosen two behaviors that promote disease, not health. Begin to notice how many times a day you choose to promote health and how many times you choose to promote disease. The purpose of this is not for you to feel guilty; the purpose is for you to begin the first step in changing any behavior—*awareness of your chosen behavior.*

We certainly are creatures of habit. Habits are automatic, nonthinking behaviors. Remember the first step in changing a habit is to become aware you are choosing a certain way of behaving.

Taking charge of your health is one of the important guidelines in the wellness philosophy. You must be actively involved in your own well-being, choosing healthy ways until they become habits. Habits take a long time to develop, so be patient. The wellness continium, depicted in Figure 2-4, shows the pathway to wellness.

Health Risk Appraisals

A new device for raising people's wellness awareness is called a health hazard appraisal or a health risk appraisal (Goetz, Duff, & Bernstein, 1980). This health promotion questionnaire looks at past and cur-

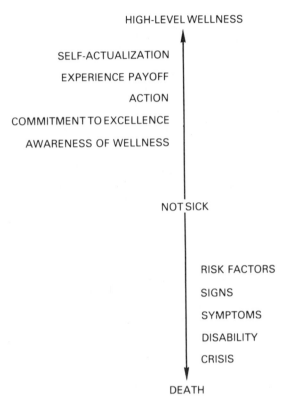

HIGH-LEVEL WELLNESS

SELF-ACTUALIZATION

EXPERIENCE PAYOFF

ACTION

COMMITMENT TO EXCELLENCE

AWARENESS OF WELLNESS

NOT SICK

RISK FACTORS

SIGNS

SYMPTOMS

DISABILITY

CRISIS

DEATH

FIGURE 2-4. This wellness diagram depicts the emerging sense of wellness as the individual moves from awareness of wellness possibilities to a state of high-level wellness. A shift needs to be made, for at present our health system basically deals with only the lower half of the continuum. There is more to health than not being sick. [Adapted from Ardell, D. *Fourteen Days to a Wellness Lifestyle.* Mill Valley, CA: Whatever Publishing, 1982.]

rent health habits, family history, and vital statistics, and then weighs you against the average in your age and race category. The results show you the average risk and your current risk with your current health-related behaviors. Your achievable risk, if you change your habits, is also given for each major category.

For example, to ascertain your health risk for the disease of cancer, your present risk with your lifestyle behaviors is compared to the average risk for getting cancer. Your risk could be .52 times the national average. In that case, your attainable risk is lower than your current risk of dying from cancer. Your health appraisal could instruct you as to what action to take to decrease your risk and increase your life expectancy to the maximum attainable.

Table 2-5
ESTIMATED PERCENTAGE CONTRIBUTION TO CAUSE
OF DEATH

Ten Leading Causes of Death	Lifestyle	Environment	Health Care Services	Biology
Heart disease	54	9	12	25
Cancer	37	24	10	29
Motor vehicle accidents	69	18	12	1
All other accidents	51	31	14	4
Stroke	50	22	7	21
Homicide	66	41	0	2
Suicide	60	35	3	2
Cirrhosis	70	9	3	18
Influenza/pneumonia	23	20	18	39
Diabetes	26	0	6	60
Total	51	19	10	20

Reprinted from *Health Self-Appraisal Report*. Washington, D.C.: The Health Corporation, 1979. With permission.

Most health appraisals take into consideration the four major factors that influence health. There is little you can do about the biological factor (e.g., your heredity and age). This factor is more or less important in diseases related to stress. The other three factors—environment, health care, and lifestyle—are to some degree under your control. Environmental factors will be more under your control when you take action: by being kinder to our planet and by supporting groups that are working to change pollution problems you can make your contribution to a healthier environment. The cost, availability, and of course the quality of prevention and treatment services available will influence your health. Your health attitude, which affects the use of these health care services, is also measured. Finally, the area over which you have the most control—lifestyle factors—is considered. The way you treat your body with food, drugs, and exercise is assessed. All four of these factors are assessed and you are compared to other individuals to formulate your life expectancy.*

The data presented in Table 2-5 show that lifestyle has a great impact

---

*These are two of the places you can write to for computor-scored health appraisals: General Health, 1046 Potomac Street, N.W., Washington, D.C. 20007, (202) 965-4881; Institute for Personal Health, P.O. Box 57219, Washington, D.C. 20037, (202)872-5379.

on the causes of death. Lifestyle contributes over 50 percent to the cause of death in seven of the ten leading causes. Only in cancer, influenza, and diabetes does the biological factor play a significant role.

Many big businesses are now using health appraisals to get their (especially male) executives to pay attention to the over-40 syndrome of overweight, overwork, overdrinking, oversmoking, and no exercise. With follow-up on the results, these appraisals are a useful tool. They can play a part in raising awareness and in prevention of the harmful effects of lifestyle factors on the quality of life.

The function of this chapter was to raise your level of awareness of your physical signs and symptoms of stress. The second purpose was to alert you to some of the treatment and prevention strategies for your signs. In the next chapter you will explore the psychological realm as it relates to stress.

3

Psychological Strategies: Choosing Your Mental Response Patterns

HOW THE MIND CREATES STRESS

To cope effectively with stress, you must consider your feelings and act rationally. For example, you do not allow yourself to yell at patients, students, or staff over their lateness. Although you have a right to be angry at repeated lateness, you fulfill your responsibility to uphold the policy standards and deal assertively with latecomers. The psychological strategies to deal with stress are based on being able to choose your response to situations that occur in your life, instead of automatically reacting.

It is important to remember that stress is not what happens to you, but the way you take what happens to you. For one nurse a difficult problem may be exciting and a challenge, whereas another nurse may find it terrifying and a threat. Your interpretation of an event determines whether you experience stress.

The perceptual and cognitive functions of your brain determine how you perceive an event. Suppose, for example, it is time for your evaluation. Your boss walks by, does not say hello, and then you get a call that he or she would like to see you for your evaluation. The way you interpret these events could create an anticipatory stress rection—if you think they mean your boss is displeased with you. If you take these events to mean the boss must be preoccupied with last minute evaluations, you would not experience stress. Your choice of response to any event depends on what you perceive and how you interpret the meaning of your perception.

Your perception of your patients, colleagues, and doctors affects how you relate to this. If you see doctors as unfeeling, your colleagues as passive, and the hemorrhoid patient as demanding, then you will relate to them with those adjective screening your incoming data. Since you tend to screen out all data that do not fit "your descriptive adjectives," you begin to make certain decisions about these people based on your perception of them through these screens. What you allow yourself to perceive depends on your senses and on your frame of reference; how you interpret the data depends on your value system and your cognitive processes. Cognitive processes involve thinking, decision making, and problem solving.

It is important to recognize how stress affects your thinking and any consequent emotional upsets. Each person's problem-solving ability is affected differently by different stresses. The problem-solving process is typically the same for everyone, however, each person experiences difficulty at different steps when stress enters the picture.

NORMAL PROBLEM-SOLVING APPROACH

Five steps are involved in the normal process of problem solving:

1. You perceive a problem. Using your senses of sight, sound, smell, taste, and touch, plus your intuitive sense, you recognize that there is a block to moving toward a goal you have decided on. Whether the goal is relevant, obtainable, or worthwhile is discussed in Chapter 7. The goal could be crossing the street in New York City or deciding on appropriate discipline for an absent staff member. The point is that you experience a problem or block in attaining your goal.

2. You begin to think. Using the cognitive processes of comparing, analyzing, monitoring, and others, you begin to figure out how to get over, under, through, or around the block. The amount and type of information you use is defined by your value system and your ability to think clearly. The amount of time you spend thinking about the problem depends on the time you have available and how important the problem seems to you. Improving the quality of your thinking is discussed later.

3. You decide on a solution. Taking all the information you have gathered into consideration, you compare alternatives based on their consequences, and you choose the best solution. (You may begin to see the silliness of "Monday morning quarterbacking" any of your decisions. Looking back over decisions and saying what you could have done is a way to make yourself feel bad, but it is hardly relevant to problem solving. The truth is that you made the best decision you could at *that* point in time when you made the decision.)

4. You take action on a solution. The action you decide upon
may be overt, or your solution may involve nonaction on your part.
For instance, you may decide to postpone taking action because timing
can be important in having people listen to you and support your
decision. Many nurses have learned that Monday mornings and Friday
afternoons are not the times to ask supervisors for time off or to
present them with problems. Delaying action in this case is a well
thought out decision. Sometimes, however, nonaction is labeled as pas-
sivity, procrastination, or passive aggressiveness. Although it is sometimes an appropriate solution, at other times you may not be taking
action because you are afraid of something—such as failure, rejection,
or disapproval. The material presented in this chapter will help you
identify what you are afraid of so that your unconscious fears will not
hamper your actions.

5. You evaluate your solution. You decide what aspects of your
solution worked and what aspects did not work. Was your timing off, or
is there never a good time? Did you need more information, or did you
overcollect information? Perhaps you need to learn more effective ways
of doing or saying something. It is important to acknowledge your successes and learn from your failures.

When you feel stressed, this seemingly straightforward problem-solving process does not flow easily. Under stress there is emotional interfer-
ence that can fog your perceptions, confuse your thinking, or paralyze
you into inaction. Perception, thinking, and action are each addressed
separately in this chapter.

When stress affects your thinking your perception can become dis-
turbed. As a nurse you have probably experienced the distortion of time
that occurs when you are working long hours. You may distort the
importance of patient problems by minimizing or maximizing the problem situation. Your perception affects your professional judgment —
therefore, some understanding of perception and the ways it interacts
with stress is important.

PERCEPTION PRINCIPLES

Table 3-1 is a list of principles of perception. These principles profoundly affect your perception and thus your stress response. Ponder
them for a few minutes.

As you can see, there are a number of variables affecting why you
see, hear, and experience what you do. These variables also affect your
behavior. For instance, if your self-image is low, you would be likely to
interpret criticism more harshly than if your self-image were high. Your

Table 3-1
PERCEPTION PRINCIPLES

No two people see things the same way.
A person's self-image influences how he or she sees the world.
A person's image of the other colors his or her relationship with the other.
A person sees things in terms of his or her own past experiences.
A person sees things differently at different times.
A person learns to see things as he or she does.
A person sees things in terms of his or her own values.
A person tends to see things largely as they were seen before.
A person sees what he or she wants to see.
A person's feelings color what he or she sees.
A person tends to complete those things which appear to be incomplete.
A person tends to either simplify or complicate those things that are not understood.
A person first sees an object as a general pattern, then focuses attention on a particular part of it.
A person tends to remember the first and last items in a series of things.
A person learns new perceptions only through new experiences.

Reprinted from Kolivosky, M. E., & Taylor, L. J. *Why do you see it that way? Principles of perception: Most applicable principles for guidelines in interpersonal relationships.* Hillsdale, Mich: Hillsdale College, 1972, p. 12. With permission

behavior would be defensive, since the criticism would be threatening to your already low self-esteem. Your image of yourself affects how you relate to others.

Unsatisfactory relationships with others are a major source of stress. Therefore, becoming aware of how your perceptions of yourself and others create communication problems is an important stress reduction technique. Begin to notice peoples' different perceptions. Notice how your own perceptions vary with your moods. Needing to be "right" in your perceptions of others is often the cause of communication difficulties.

Finally, perceptions are the mainspring of motivation. If you have not completed a nursing assignment, your attention will return to this incompletion. Your focus on this incompletion will function as a motivator for you to complete the assignment. Not completing assignments or not finishing projects leads to an increase in your stress level: it is difficult to deal with the present when your mind is focused on the past or future.

Your perception process is thus affected by numerous other variables in addition to stress. Thinking about a problem is a complex process that begins with perception and leads to a decision. During times of stress your mind may become confused or distracted, and this process is interfered with. Many errors in thinking are a consequence of stress affecting the normal thought processes.

ERRORS IN THINKING

Albert Ellis, the founder of a theory and therapy called rational emotive therapy, describes several common errors in thinking (Ellis & Harper, 1979):

1. Dichotomous thinking. "I either work or stay home." This is either/or, black/white thinking. Your mind naturally does either/or thinking when you initially think about a problem, but then you usually think further. People who operate basically in this mode are seen as inflexible. Under stress you attempt to screen out stimuli, and this type of thinking accomplishes just that.

2. Reliance on another's judgment "What *you* think about me or what *you* think is the right answer is more important than what I think." Sometimes this type of thinking is useful when dealing with authoritative types—such as policemen. Otherwise, recognize that others may dislike you or not agree with you for completely irrational reasons (e.g., because you remind them of someone). If "what will they think of me?" runs your life, you will be especially interested in the section "Guilt," later on in this chapter.*

3. Overgeneralizing. "All doctors are egomaniacs." "Nursing is a dead-end street." "University hospitals are the only place to work." Overgeneralizations are vague and indefinite statements. The hospital looks very different when you think all doctors do the best they can, rather than generalize negatively about them.

4. Stereotyping. "Pediatric nurses all love children." "Psychiatric nurses are all neurotic." Both of these statements create mental pictures. Stereotyping is fixing an image, either positive or negative, in your mind. "Category *X* persons are . . ." is the standard form of stereotyping. By stereotyping you divide the world into categories, and each of these categories has a permanent set of qualities or characteristics. In the end you respond to the category, not to the individual or the situation. For instance, create a picture of a "hippie," a "drug user," and a "feminist"; each of these words create images in your mind. It is a very convenient way to deal with the world—you do not have to think. The next time you meet a drug user you believe you already know about people who fall in that category, so you do not spend time thinking about that individual.

---

*Remember also—"Anyone who is always worrying about what other people think of them would be surprised to know how seldom people do" (John C. Vivian).

Ellis does not say this, but I think stereotyping leads to overgeneralizing. Make vague, indefinite statements about someone or something long enough and you begin to believe yourself.

5. *Catastrophizing.* "The new intern did not say hello this morning—I have been erased from his mind." "This day has started badly—the whole day will be terrible." Catastrophizing is viewing events as 100 percent bad.

These errors in your thinking raise your stress level because effective problem solving cannot be conducted in the presence of unclear thinking. Your perception and your interpretation of events play a large role in coping with stress. Begin to notice how you perceive events, without a right/wrong attitude, and you will begin to unblock your perceptual apparatus. Observe yourself as you launch off into one of your erroneous thinking patterns. The way to change these patterns is to become aware, stop your pattern when you notice it, and change it to a thinking pattern that focuses on the present situation and your present needs. This is not to say that long-term consequences are to be ignored in your thinking; they are indeed to be factored into your consideration.

PSYCHOLOGICAL SIGNS AND SYMPTOMS OF STRESS

Psychological signs and symptoms are a result of ineffective handling of one's emotions and distorted thinking patterns. Table 3-2 is a listing of signs; write down any you have experienced in the past six months. Notice whether any of these signs and symptoms are increasing, and place an "X" next to those. Circle the ones that are of most concern for you today. Contemplate.

ANXIETY AS A STRESS SYMPTOM

Anxiety is the most prominent symptom involved in stress reactions and psychosomatic disorders. When the individual experiences the signs of anxiety he or she often is unable to think clearly and is emotionally troubled. Symptoms of anxiety are often associated with other psychological illnesses such as depression and dissociation.

Anxiety is not in itself pathological, and to a certain extent it is unavoidable. Anxiety is considered normal when its intensity and character are appropriate in a given situation (Freud, 1936; May, 1950). A person is more alert, sensitive, and perceptive to a situation when moder-

Table 3-2
EMOTIONAL AND MENTAL SIGNS AND SYMPTOMS OF
STRESS

Emotional	Intellectual
Irritability, overreaction to some relatively minor situation	Forgetfulness, preoccupation
	Blocking
Angry outbursts, short-tempered reactions, hostility	Increased fantasy life
	Decreased concentration, especially on complicated jobs
Jealousy	Inattention to detail
Lack of interest, withdrawn, apathetic, cannot get up in the morning	Past- rather than present-oriented
	Decreased creativity
Crying tendencies	Slower thinking, slower reactions, difficulty learning subjects
Blaming others, suspicious attitude	"Couldn't care less" attitude,
Self-deprecating	mentally lazy, inclined to path of
Diminished initiative	least resistance
Reduction of personal involvement with others	
Depression, worrying	
Negative attitude, cynical	
Job dissatisfaction	

ately anxious. People actually seek the tension rise through movies, carnivals, spy novels, and competitive sports. The key is that the anxiety must not be too intense or last too long.

The type of anxiety discussed in this chapter is not the pleasure of excitement, but the nervous tension you experience as you are responding to a threat. The threat, real or imagined, can be a source of intolerable tension to your mind and body. Your body may feel electrified with tension or tied in knots as your muscles contract for fight or flight. Whatever the "weak link" is in your body, it is likely to begin to break down under this pressure. In the last chapter you identified your body vulnerabilities; in this chapter the focus is on your cognitive and emotional vulnerabilities.

You experience anxiety when you see a need for a defensive position against a threat. The anxious preparation often takes the form of rehearsing the anticipated danger so that when it finally materializes you have already organized your defense in advance. Janis (1958) reports that this is an important factor in preparation for surgery. As a nurse, you are surely able to remember many instances in which momentary anticipation served to protect you against being overwhelmed by a sense of helplessness.

Psychological symptoms occur when you do become overwhelmed to some degree by the anxiety. When there is no adequate justification for it, when it is exaggerated or unduly prolonged, or when it gives rise to defensive maneuvers that interfere seriously with the enjoyment and the effectiveness of your life, then the anxiety is considered pathological (Cameron, 1963). If the anxiety is diffused in hyperactivity or is repressed and you lose spontaneity, then anxiety is seen as pathological. Impulsive acts, sexual or aggressive, are also seen as distortions of unbearable anxiety. All these behaviors represent some disorganization of your personality and interpersonal relationship.

Plainly said, when you are afraid you will experience some degree of anxiety. You may or may not know what you are afraid of. In either case, the degree of tension you experience determines your level of anxiety. If, in reading the preceding paragraph you noted that some of the characteristics described apply to you, then begin to take seriously the need to understand the sources of your anxiety and reduce the level of your stress responses.

Anxiety can be manifested in your thinking in one of three ways. Your mind feels as if it is racing—thoughts stream by so quickly you cannot concentrate on any one of them. Second, your mind selects a thought and tries to follow it, and all of a sudden you cannot seem to compelte the thought sequence. Your mind has reached a dead end, and either you cannot come to a conclusion or the conclusion does not seem sensible. This is called confusion. The third way your mind behaves under stress is to go blank. You were thinking (and sometimes you were talking), and all of a sudden, nothing—no words. Often much to your embarrassment, you lose your train of thought and your mind is blank.

Whether you mind races, you get confused, or you go blank, anxiety is affecting your thinking. Each of these signs can be both a cause and an effect of stress.

DISSOCIATION: A MEANS TO COPE WITH ANXIETY

Dissociation results from an attempt to isolate something that causes anxiety. This adaptive attempt to escape anxiety carries with it a sense of estrangement from objects, places, persons, or self. You have probably had this experience several times in your life and have not realized it was call a dissociative reaction. For instance, remember a time when you received catastrophic news or something terrible happened. In order to keep your emotions within manageable limits, you distanced yourself from the incident and probably felt unreal or that what you were witnessing was not really happening.

When these mild, transient experiences become more intense, last longer, or escape your control, then the dissociation becomes abnormal. Barbara Gordon, who wrote the 1979 best-seller *I'm Dancing as Fast as I*

Can, described her depersonalization experience vividly: "There's a sense of being glassy, something separates us . . . I really feel like there is a little Saran Wrap around me, and in order to reach you I have to poke out . . . you feel like glass and you bump into things because you can't feel your edges" (Polak, 1981). Ms. Gordon has described one side of the dissociative experience.

You may think, "Why should I see this definition in a stress book?" It is because I have seen a number of cases of dissociation that originated from an increase in job stress. One woman was involved in an automobile accident, one was picked up for shoplifting (kleptomania), and one found herself in Miami. All of these women did not pay attention to the first occurrence of dissociation, and one did not take note of the second occurrence. Once all three saw the relationship of their behavior to stress, there was a lifting of their depression. None has had any incidents in the past year. Freud's anxiety is today's stress, and both cause dissociation.

If you have diagnosed psychiatric problems in the neurotic or psychotic categories, you need to monitor your stress levels closely, just as if you had diabetes and were monitoring your sugar, or had myocardial infarction and were monitoring your electrocardiograms. Everyone's psychic system can tolerate only so much overload. Some people's bodies break down under stress, and for some people the vulnerable area is their mind.

It is important you know *your* system's limits. There are many nursing situations that can tax your limits. Dealing with doctors, staff, and patients can all be stressful at times. For instance, it is important to remember that it matters little if your nurse colleagues on the night shift think Mr. Jones is adorable, if for some reason he upsets *you.* Know he upsets you and deal as little as you can with him until you figure out why he upsets you. Then decide how you can best cope with him. As long as he is getting good nursing care, your responsibility is fulfilled. After all, the fact is you are not going to like all patients.

UNDERSTANDING AND COPING
WITH EMOTIONS

Understanding and accepting your responses to situations in life is the first step in treating psychological burnout. The second step is to recognize the methods that work best to keep your mind in a more relaxed state. The third is to consistently and repeatedly practice the workable methods. Remember that treating psychological burnout, i.e., changing mental response patterns, is a lifelong learning process—a process that requires having patience with yourself.

Remember that the stress response is actually the fight or flight response, involving the feelings of anger and fear. Anger and fear are legitimate feelings to have. As you were growing up you needed to receive permission to feel these feelings and to learn appropriate ways to express them. If you did not receive that permission or education, you are likely to have difficulty today.

Anger and Fear

In our culture it is less permissible for men to show fear and for women to show anger. Many times this is reinforced by our families— "you shouldn't be mad at your brother," or later, in nursing school, "there is nothing to be afraid of Mr. Rose, you are only giving your first injection." I have never understood how "don't worry" and "you shouldn't be afraid" can be thought of as supportive statements. They only make you feel inadequate or guilty for feeling what you feel. Healthy expressions of anger and fear need to be supported to keep communication channels open.

Anger is that emotion which accompanies the realization that someone or something is not changing in accord with your desires. Perhaps you think of anger as caused by others' self-centered, stupid, and inconsiderate actions; the truth is that *you* are creating your anger. Your feeling results from the meaning you give to the event, not from the event itself.

Feeling a feeling is not the same as acting on a feeling. Many times you may feel anger because of how you interpret a situation; however, you can begin to take control of your emotions by not acting on your anger. Aggression does not equal anger. Violence does not equal anger. There is a difference between feeling a feeling, expressing a feeling, and acting on a feeling. A healthy statement about anger from a parent would be "I see you feel angry. You may tell your baby brother. You may not hit him." The admonition "you should not feel angry" only switches the feeling of anger at baby brother to guilt, which is simply anger at self. The statement "you shouldn't feel X" triggers you to feel guilty for feeling X.

Fear is an emotion accompanying the contemplation of the unknown. Fear is often described as anxiety felt in the presence of danger. The danger is perceived as a threat to your emotional or physical survival. What scares you, again, varies with what your internal thoughts tell you about a situation or person. The extremes of fear—terror and panic—are overwhelming feelings that can paralyze you or lead to frantic, aimless activity.

People are conditioned to fear certain situations. Having a mother and then a nervous nursing instructor constantly saying, "be careful," leads to nervous tension when this thought is repeated internally. Likewise, if either of these people is given to attacking you verbally in emotional outbursts, you learn to live in fear of these fits. When a patient takes a turn for the worse you may feel scared. When you have a new responsibility or role you have never performed you may feel scared. When you are confronted with an unknown situation or a new person, one of the emotions that you could manifest is fear. Later you will begin to identify fear-producing situations for yourself.

Identifying what triggers your anger and fear reactions is an important part of learning to control your stress response. Since these are the feelings most often associated with the fight or flight response, having control over them allows you to have choices over your response to stressors.

Begin by identifying three things that anger you in your work climate and three in your personal life. Ask yourself "What could someone else do that would be guaranteed to anger me? What would make me mad (whether or not I show it)? Write down your answers.

For each of your six responses, answer the following:

1. Is this a behavior you feel angry at yourself for doing when *you* occasionally do it? (It is uncomfortable to see people doing what you do because it reminds you of your own fallible nature.)
2. Is this a behavior you never do and you feel others should not do either? Are you self-righteous about not doing it? (Many self-righteous individuals are converts. They used to do or be that way and are not now. Sometimes people who have never had any experience, or have no sense of being able to empathize with what it may be like to be in that situation, assume a self-righteous attitude.)

Once you identify the experience that makes you angry and begin to see which of the two above reasons triggers you into creating your upset, then it is time to ask some more self-awareness generating questions. For example, what are you telling yourself about the situation? Maybe you say, "He should be more considerate of his patients." Perhaps you say to yourself, "She doesn't care about us as staff, she is only interested in covering the floors, not in good patient care." What pictures do you create in your mind that reinforce your anger? A picture of the other floor nurses who called in sick relaxing at home while you are doing the work for two would foster anger. Maybe you picture the supervisor relaxing as you are running about doing patient care. What you tell yourself about the situation and the images you visualize help maintain your anger response.

The next time you feel angry at someone, take time to look at yourself and see if you are looking at your negative behavior or if you are engaging in self-righteous anger. Next, take note of how you reinforce your anger with what you tell yourself and what images you create. If you can repeatedly observe your own behavior you will begin to understand and change your internal, and therefore your external, response.

Often it is difficult to convince people of the importance of modifying their anger responses because they feel so justified in their anger. Persuading yourself to stop indulging in anger responses and instead trying to understand how you create your anger by your internal thoughts is no easy task. You can take charge of your stress response by developing an awareness of what triggers your reactions.

Observing your own anger responses is an ongoing assignment for you. Its purpose is to learn about yourself, not to feel guilty. Guilt occurs because you judge yourself with respect to what you have or have not done; guilt does not occur when you watch yourself. Guilt stops you from thinking and learning, because you are focusing on your mind chatter, rather than problem solving.

The same is true for many of your fear responses. Begin the process by identifying what scares you. You can choose to avoid certain people or situations. You limit yourself with your fears if you choose to use avoidance as your major coping technique. Write down five things you do not do because you are afraid. A few examples may be going back to school, asserting yourself with your head nurse and/or doctor, or possibly giving up sugar or coffee. All these involve some change in behavior that can trigger the fear response.

In understanding your fear you need to remember that it is a protective response each of us has. To make a change you must look at what you really are afraid of and what support you will need to face the fear. In order to understand your fear further, do the following exercise. Picture one of the situations that you are fearful of and answer the following questions:

1. What is scaring you—fear of failure, rejection? What are you afraid of?
2. What are you afraid of if your fear becomes true?
3. If that happens, what are you afraid of?
4. Then if that happens, what are you afraid of?

Continue this line of questioning until nothing more comes to your mind. It is important that you begin to understand the root of your fear so that you can take steps to reduce the amount of your fear. For example, going to talk to your dean or supervisor because you are dissatisfied in your work can create anxiety. Believing they will fire you or yell and scream at you could arouse fears strong enough to paralyze you. (Both of these outcomes are possible, but not probable.) Your fear of speaking up may be basically a fear of criticism or a fear of losing control when criticized. Once you have identified your fear you can develop skills in a step-by-step process that can greatly reduce your fears.

Another example is a fear of working with Mr. Moses, a terminal cancer patient. Here again, being afraid could probably lead you to avoid learning more about dealing with a dying patient. You could reduce your fear with more knowledge about death and dying. However, is this the real issue? Perhaps this would only be treating a symptom of the problem. The real fear of your own mortality may be the issue. Learning to cope with your own mortality may be the real help you need. A week with Dr. Kubler-Ross can help greatly.* Perhaps you could begin by doing some reading (Garfield, 1979; Kubler-Ross, 1969, 1974; O'Conner, 1976); perhaps contemplating, or talking with a friend would be helpful.

Identifying your anger and your fear triggers will help you gain some degree of control over your emotions. Three other emotions are discussed below: disappointment, hurt, and guilt. All three involve some unfulfilled expectation of self or of another. You can gain control over these emotional experiences also.

Disappointment

Disappointment, according to *Webster's,* is the feeling of being made unhappy by the failure of one's hopes or expectations. It is the feeling you feel when you plan for or hope for something to occur and it does not occur because of your or another's lack of effort, or perhaps just fate. Most often your disappointment comes not because others have failed to keep their promises, but because your expectations of yourself and of other are different from your/their performance.

Disappointment over foiled plans is a common emotional experience. An alternative to sitting and sulking over a disappointment is to decide "OK, now what?" The key to treating disappointment is to look at your choices. For instance, you lost your weekend off because of short staffing—you can sulk, or you can see what you can do for yourself that is nurturing and fun.

Since disappointment arises from expectations, and an expectation is presuming that an event will occur, having reasonable expectations is a sure-fire way to reduce disappointment. Reasonable expectations would not include perfectionism or mind reading on the part of others. Perhaps you know nurses who are almost always in a state of disappointment because of their belief in fortune telling. They continually visualize in

---

*For information on workshops on death and dying contact Dr. Elizabeth Kubler-Ross, Shanti Nilaye, P.O. Box 2396, Escondido, CA 92025.

their minds how they want their work and personal life to be and do not take action to create the desired situation expecting it to "just happen." Expecting others to know your needs is like expecting them to be capable of mind reading. In reality, people are basically too occupied with the running of their own lives to mind read. To expect them to is setting yourself up for disappointment and hurt.

Instead, identify your wants and ask for what you want. Let the experience of getting without asking be the icing on the cake, not the cake. Learn that imagining and hoping are not equivalent to planning and acting assertively. The former often lead to disappointment, as may the latter; however, planning and acting create some sense of control over life and asking often increases your chances of getting. What will you ask for today? What will you plan for today?

Hurt

Hurt, like disappointment, often arises out of unfulfilled expectations. "I feel hurt because she didn't show appreciation for the fact that I worked overtime." "I feel hurt because Dr. Jones didn't believe that I carried out his order." Each of these statements has a built-in set of expectations that the other person should have behaved differently.

To hurt is to cause physical or emotional injury, damage, or pain to another. Hurt is often thought of in relation to wounding someone's feelings. These definitions view hurt as generated by another person. In truth, hurt is self-generated mental distress. Reducing your self-made hurts will greatly help you deal with the harm (intentional or unintentional) from others.

I see hurt as a combination of anger and sadness. Often it involves anger at feeling taken advantage of, abused in some way, or treated unfairly by someone of importance. The sadness is connected to the loss of trust that accompanies being hurt. Most of the time the hurt needs to be acknowledged and dealt with in order for the trust to be reestablished. If not dealt with, the hurt festers unresolved. Festering hurt creates stress and destroys relationships as years of accumulated hurt create resentment.

The hurt created from broken agreements and broken promises needs to be acknowledged, as well as the hurt that occurs when we are not treated with consideration. Stating "I felt hurt when you didn't keep your promise," will help reduce the stress of unfinished business. Clearly verblizing the hurt feeling begins the process of resolving emotional conflicts.

The hurt that comes from unfulfilled hopes and expectations often can be dealt with internally. It is important not to get into blaming others with the standard reaction, "You should have known I felt . . . I wanted . . . I expected. . . ." When you expect people to "mind read" your hopes and your expectations, you are setting yourself up to feel hurt. The clear expression of your needs will reduce hurt feelings in these circumstances. Doing this will go a long way to reduce the damage you could create in your relationships if you blame others.

Guilt

Guilt is the feeling you experience when you have done "wrong" according to some legal or ethical value system. Not living up to your expectations of yourself and not acting according to your value system creates guilt. You experience guilt when there is a discrepancy between what you think you should do and what you have done. The distance between your ideal self and your real self (who you are now) determines your degree of guilt. The closer you are to who you think you should be, the less anxiety and guilt you will experience. You have the choice to change who you are or to change who you think you should be (your value system). Guilt can be abated through a process of closing the gap between who you think you should be and who you are now (Horney, 1945).

Albert Ellis (Ellis & Harper, 1979) relates guilt to Horney's "tryanny of the shoulds," in his ideas about self-stressing. He sees guilt as a consequence of telling yourself you are bad for not doing what you ought to have done. This is especially important to remember around the issue of patients dying. Nurses have essentially the same range of reactions to death as lay people: the more unexpected the event, the more difficult it is to deal with. While we share our emotions of grief and loss with others over the event, when a patient dies we often add on guilt.

> The guilt is caused by the persistent idea (no matter how progressive we are, no matter how hard we try to purge it, it is still lurking there in some dark corner of our preconscious) that we can defeat death. So every time a patient dies a small voice from within informs me that if only I had tried harder, or intervened sooner, or knew more, that person would still be alive. (Pines, 1981, p. 9)

That voice needs to be dealt with, otherwise you will torture yourself. Perhaps talking to your oncology or hospice nurse colleagues would help, since their job many times is to help a patient die.

It is important to learn the difference between rightful and unreasonable expectations of yourself. Ask yourself two questions: Why do I feel guilty? Should I feel guilty?

Most of you need to reappraise the rules that you have set down for yourselves. Take a look at the principles you use to guide your life. Are they truly yours or are they prescriptions of parents, friends, and society?

Ellis suggests that you establish your own guidelines to help you distinguish between reasonable and unreasonable demands you place on yourself.

Other psychologists have called this the internal dialogue or self-talk. When everything you say to yourself about yourself is negative, you believe you deserve to feel guilty. If you congratulate yourself for your successes and treat your mistakes as learning experiences, then your self-talk will be more positive. Positive self-talk is one technique that warrants further discussion.

"I am what I think I am," is the simple basis for the idea of positive self-talk. Saying to myself, "I am stupid," which is exactly the same thing as thinking I am stupid, will create a self-image of stupidity. I may then behave stupidly in fulfillment of this self-image. Through self-talk you can become what you tell yourself you are; you can become what you think you are. (However, as stated by Norman Vincent Peale, "Never forget the basic fact about yourself—you are greater and finer than you think you are.")

This concept of negative self-talk can also be applied to a group of people, such as the nursing profession: "We don't have the power to change the administration, the power to make a difference in how this country's health care system works. No, we are powerless. There is nothing we can do." This negative self-talk as a group is perpetuated when each of you gives up trying to make a difference. Being willing to stand up and be heard comes from positive self-talk. Sound like a political rally? Perhaps it is—a rallying call for each nurse to take charge of personal and professional power by changing the way he or she thinks about self-image.

Worry

Worry is another term for this self-talk strategy. Worry is thinking about and feeling anxious over some event that could be a catastrophe. This future event looks like a potential tragedy now. What you repeatedly forget is that it is never as bad as you thought it would be when you actually experience this potential tragedy. Moreover, how many of these tragedies did you plan for that never occurred? All that wasted strategizing self-talk depletes your energy and makes you anxious.

Imagine what you could have done with all that time—those sunsets, beautiful flowers, and close times with a friend you missed. When you are off worrying how to prevent your adolescent daughter from getting pregnant or how to deal with Surgeon Ego you are missing a lot. I am not against planning—Chapter 7 is devoted to it. Worrying and planning are not the same. *Continuous* strategic planning is not necessary. When you develop an attitude that you can handle almost anything that happens—a pregnant adolescent or a screaming doctor—you will begin to worry less. Your control lies in controlling your response to situations, not the other person.

FOUR METHODS FOR DECREASING NEGATIVE SELF-TALK

Worry, like the experience of guilt, is a negative self-talk pattern. They both are guaranteed to make you feel uncomfortable and feel bad about yourself. They can be replaced with positive feelings by doing the following:

- Steadily increasing your belief that you can control your emotional responses, not external events
- Increasing your wisdom about the difference between what you can control and what you cannot
- Knowing, perhaps redefining, and living according to your values
- Setting time aside each day to do planning for your day, as well as your life.

These four measures require certain skills that you will need to master. A few of these skills are mentioned in the discussion of each below.

Controlling Your Emotional Response

Controlling your emotional response requires that you first know your emotional triggers. You have already begun to do this with the anger and fear exercises. Make a list of the types of scenes (e.g., your relief is late) and the types of people (e.g., arrogant) that upset you. These scenes and types of people act as triggers to your emotional state.

Dealing with emotional upsets involves recognizing the triggering person or event, followed by knowing what you tell yourself about the occurrence (self-talk). For instance, dealing with someone who has a false sense of self-importance may be upsetting only after you call that person arrogant. When you get emotionally upset, first look at yourself—not to find fault, but to truly understand what upsets you. Having identified your upset, begin changing your self-talk, determine what your options are for remedying the situation, then take the best choice and act. Remember that first you must identify what you are telling yourself about the situation or person; listen to your self-talk and change it to helpful, supportive talk.

A skill useful here is assertiveness. Using the following simple formula will help you control your response: "I feel X, when you do Y, because of *Z*, and what I'd like instead is [request behavior change]." For the late relief nurse it would take the form, "I feel upset when you come to work 15 minutes late because now I will miss my train: I would like you to be on time." For dealing with the arrogant person, name the behavior that disturbs you. Do not say, "I feel angry when you are arrogant . . . "; the *X* part needs to name the behavior, not judge it. The assertive communication paradigm is thus a three-part assertion message:

1. A nonjudgmental description of the behavior to be changed;
2. A disclosure of the assertor's feelings and a clarification of the concrete and tangible effect of the other person's behavior on the assertor;
3. A statement of the desired behavior change.

The last segment of this approach may be simply to talk about the behavior; you may also request the person to think about the consequences of his or her behavior. The "I'd like . . . " part of your statement informs the person of your preferences. You may choose to delete this part until you have heard the other person's response to your assertive statement.

Unfortunately, sending an assertive messages does not guarantee that the other person will respond positively to your request. Even the best sent message is likely to trigger a defensive response because often the person feels threatened. People feel uncomfortable being told that they have a negative effect on others.

The six-step process presented in Table 3-3 will help you cope with the stress of dealing with defensiveness. This process was designed to reduce the escalation of agression and its destructiveness in communication. The process is meant to act as a guideline for handling defensiveness. A more detailed description of the process is given by Bolton (1979, pp. 159–175).

Knowing What You Can and Cannot Control

It is easier to decide whether or not you can control something if you have effective and efficient problem-solving and decision-making skills. You would then control what you can in the present situation and do preventive planning for the future. Frustration is the result of trying to change the unchangeable or trying the same method repeatedly with hopes that this time it will work.

People can change only from the inside out—you cannot change another person. Your own changing will certainly affect other people and then they may change. It is important to remember that when your goal is to change them you had better be ready for your plan to backfire, be-

Table 3-3
SIX-STEP ASSERTION PROCESS FOR DEALING WITH
PREDICTABLE DEFENSIVE RESPONSES

I. *Preparation*
   A. Write the message before sending it to diffuse some of your pent-up feelings.
   B. Test the appropriateness of your message.
      1. Do not trespass on the other's space.
      2. The issue is a persistent concern.
      3. Are you likely to get your needs met?
   C. Rehearse the interaction.
   D. Secure an appointment to talk.
   E. Take the timing into consideration.

II. *Sending the message*
   A. Do not begin with small talk.
   B. Use body language congruent with the message, do not appear ambivalent; the elements of body language include eye contact, posture, gestures, facial expressions, and voice.

III. *Being silent*

IV. *Reflectively listening to the other's defensive response*
   A. Shifting back and forth between listening and assertion several times accomplishes the following:
      1. It diminishes the other's defensiveness.
      2. What you learn by listening modifies your need to continue your assertion.
      3. You may find that a strong need of the other person conflicts with your need: use collaborative problem solving.
      4. You learn how the other person perceives you and your relationship.
   B. Examples of reflective listening responses are:
      1. "You feel that I don't understand."
      2. "You think I should pay more attention to your needs."
      3. "If I understand you, you see the situation differently."
   C. Handle hostile responses.
      1. Reflect the other person's content and feelings, with special emphasis on feelings.
      2. Limit your interaction to an assertion message and reflective listening—*no sidetracking.*
      3. Treat the other person with respect.
         a. Keep your voice free of sarcasm or condescension.
         b. Do not use judgmental words.
      4. Reassert your original assertion message.
   D. Deal with questions.
      1. Do not answer the question.
      2. Reply with a reflective listening response.

E. Sidestep debates.
   1. Watch out for the other person taking a defensive position and using mental quickness and verbal ability to win when the person "doesn't have a leg to stand on."
   2. Refuse to debate by giving a reflective listening response.
F. Cope with tears.
   1. Be aware this is a manipulative way to dodge confrontation and change.
   2. Reflect upon what the other person is sad about and then gently reaffirm.
   3. If the other person is very upset stop the conversation and continue it at a specific time later that day or the next day.
G. Overcome withdrawal
   1. Total silence and a poker face indicate the person is uncomfortable and defensive.
   2. Provide a lot of silence, reflect what body language is saying, then reassert.
   3. If the person remains silent say, "I take your silence to mean that you don't want to talk about it and that you will meet my needs by [doing what behavior change you are requesting]."
H. Help the other person express understanding of your predicament and/or a solution to the problem; catch the slightest nuance of an offered solution.

V. *Recycling the process*
A. Typically, it takes three to ten repetitions of the assertion message to change the other's behavior.
B. If you reach a stalemate, increase the effect of the feeling comunicated by your tone of voice and body language.
C. Be sincere—express neither more nor less emotion than you feel.
D. Maintain a balance between rational control systems and genuine expression of emotion.*

VI. *Focusing on the solution*
A. Do not back the person into a corner.
B. The process of reconciliation makes your relationship stronger.
C. Accept only a solution that meets your needs.
D. Do not insist the other person be cheerful about meeting your needs.
E. Paraphrase the solution back to the other.
F. Say "thanks."
G. Arrange a time when you will check with each other to make sure the solution is working.

---

*As theologian Revel Howe has noted, "Crisis in dialogue occurs when the participants . . . fail really to address each other but turn away defensively, each within himself, for the purposes of self-justification" (Howe, 1963, p. 84).

Adapted from Bolton R. *People Skills*. Englewood Cliffs, NJ, Prentice-Hall, 1979, pp. 159–175.

cause people do not like being manipulated. Your time is better spent changing what you can; stress results from the frustration of unsuccessful change attempts.

Frustration is the awareness that whatever goal you planned to attain you are not going to reach it. Feeling frustrated is usually the result of having tried several times for the same goal. The frustration is stronger the more significant the goal is. The question that always follows the feeling of frustration is, "Shall I try again?" The answers to that question and the subsequent question—"How shall I try again?"—play a significant role in determining your stress level. If your plans are met with resistance many times, then rather than accept failure, take time to check two things.

First check to see if your goals are realistic and if the strategy allows for imperfections on your part and on the part of others. Many times I have heard frustrated nurses cry, "If only I had thought of that," and, "It would have worked if only she would have done her part." The first comment reveals inadequate planning and the second comment speaks to the issue of inadequate follow-up. You know whether people are doing their part only if you check.

Second, check whether you are meeting with resistance because of *how* you are presenting yourself, rather than because of *what* you are presenting. You will need the feedback of a few trusted friends or colleagues. Some of you would be surprised to see how you come across to people. Whenever the opportunity avails itself, learn how you do come across to people. It is invaluable self-knowledge.

On an emotional level frustration resembles the feeling of helplessness and hopelessness, but when you feel frustration you are still fighting—you have not given up. If you keep trying long enough without the desired results, you get a feeling of helplessness. Do not allow yourself to keep trying that long. It is important to know when to throw in the towel and say, "I quit trying," whether it is in regard to your marriage or your career plan.

It is just as important to know when to stick with it and activate another strategy. You need to decide if it is worth the price you are paying in terms of stress. Because we all have different comfort zones, our degrees of tolerance vary. Check to make sure you are not suffering unnecessarily or giving up too easily.

Another way to reduce frustration is to become more flexible. Flexibility is a willingness to move in the direction of the force. The willow bends with the force of the wind and remains standing after the storm; the oak resists the force and breaks. If you believe in only *your* way and someone comes along with a different way, you are likely to feel the stress of resistance. Flexibility in your thinking will allow you to bend reasonably with the winds of change.

Frustration results when you cannot get things or people to change according to your desires. Gaining the wisdom to focus your efforts of change on yourself will increase your sense of control over your life. Chapter 7 is devoted to strategies for changing yourself.

Whether changing yourself or coping with your changing world, your view of change helps determine your stress level. This was demonstrated in a study by Oskins (1979), in which 79 ICU nurses rated 12 narratives as stressful or nonstressful and identified them as a challenge or a threat. The results showed that all 12 narratives were seen as stressful. The same events were seen as challenging by some nurses and as threatening by others. How can this be explained? The answer lies in realizing that what each person feels depends on that individual's perception and appraisal of the situation, not the situation. Stress is your response to your own interpretation of events.

Knowing, Redefining, and Living According to Your Values

How you perceive change, respond to change, or try to control change depends on your values concerning change. One of my stress survival kit tricks* to cope with this ever-changing world is to see change as an opportunity, not a crisis. This idea reflects a valuing of change as a chance to learn and grow. Clarifying your values is a skill in coping with change; it is discussed in Chapter 7. For now, begin to familiarize yourself with your values about change by noticing how you view change: Challenge or threat? Opportunity or crisis? Notice the difference in how you feel when you view change one way and when you view it the other. When you view it as a catastrophe you feel anxious; when you see it as an opportunity you feel excited and energized to action. Physiologically, anxiety and excitement are the same; your interpretation makes one unpleasant and the other pleasant.

Planning Your Life

Planning for change can do a lot to relieve worry, guilt, and frustration. Planning your day and your life does not necessarily kill spontaneity. Flexible planning allows for life's spontaneous ups and downs. Planning simply creates a structure that decreases the stress of uncertainty.

The negative self-talk patterns of worry and guilt are greatly relieved by planning. Planning allows you to focus on what is important for you and involves prioritized action strategies to accomplish your goals. Rather

---

*The concept of "survival kit" comes from Ardell (1977).

than sitting and worrying about a task, sit down, break it into manageable pieces, and develop steps to reach the good feeling of accomplishment. Your resistance to planning creates worry, as well as guilt over failures. In Chapter 7 you will examine your resistances and learn planning and organizing skills.

PERFECTIONISM

Someone who has too much of a need for planning, a low tolerance for ambiguity and uncertainty, and a passion for detail is a *perfectionist.* Perfectionism causes continually high levels of stress in an individual. The perfectionist is always on call to correct or to prevent the smallest mistake. Trying to create a perfect world around you is defying reality. To quote Cardinal Neuman, "Nothing would be done at all if you waited until you could do it so well that no one could find fault in it." Perfectionism is a contributing factor in burnout, especially among administrators. Veninga (1979) mentions three scripts that show the role of perfectionism in creating burnout: (1) Trust Only Yourself, (2) Everybody Should See the World as I See It, and (3) I'm Going to Succeed Even if It Kills Me! These scripts are the basis for how these nurses approach life. As you can imagine by their titles, they lead to high levels of stress.

Take the test in Table 3-4 to see if you fall into the category of perfectionist. This scale was developed by Burns (1980) at the University of Pennsylvania Mood Clinic. It lists a number of attitudes or beliefs that people sometimes hold. Decide how much you agree with each statement according to the following code: +2, I agree very much; +1, I agree somewhat; 0, I feel neutral about this; −1, I disagree slightly; −2, I disagree strongly. For each statement choose the number that best describes how you think most of the time. Be sure to choose only one answer for each attitude. There are no "right" or "wrong" answers, so try to respond according to the way you usually feel and behave.

To score this test, add up your scores on all items, noting that plus numbers and minus numbers cancel each other out. For example, if your answer on five items is +1 and your score on each of the other five is −1, your total test score is 0. If you answered +2 on all the items, your total score is +20, revealing a very high degree of perfectionism. If you answered −2 on every item, your score is −20, signifying a strongly nonperfectionistic mind set. Preliminary studies suggest that about one-half of the population is likely to score from +2 to +16, indicating varying degrees of perfectionism.

If you scored at the higher end then you need to pay attention to the fact that your pattern of perfectionism is stressing you. I know you will

Table 3-4
PERFECTIONISM SCALE

If I do not set the highest standards for myself, I am likely to end up a second-rate person.
People will probably think less of me if I make a mistake.
If I cannot do something really well, there is little point in doing it at all.
I should be upset if I make a mistake.
If I try hard enough, I should be able to excel at anything I attempt.
It is shameful for me to display weaknesses or foolish behavior.
I should not have to repeat the same mistake many times.
An average performance is bound to be unsatisfying to me.
Failing at something important means I am less of a person.
If I scold myself for failing to live up to my expectations, it will help me to do better in the future.

Reprinted from Burns, D. The perfectionist's script for self defeat. *Psychology Totday Magazine,* November 1980, pp. 34–52. Copyright © 1980, Ziff-Davis Publishing Company. With permission.

want to cling to your idea that the scale is useless or that for you perfectionism is not a *significant* problem. Your stubborn insistence will rob you of the awareness you need to begin to change this pattern. Perfectionists, read the next section carefully!

Knowing you are a perfectionist and even knowing the origins of your perfectionism are not sufficient for change. The first step necessary for you to change is for you to know that perfectionism is not to your advantage. Most perfectionists actually believe that perfectionism has more benefits than costs. Burns (1980) suggests you make a list of the advantages and disadvantages of perfectionism.

The second step is for you to learn you can experience a great degree of satisfaction performing in a less than outstanding manner. The all-or-nothing thinking perfectionists have leads you to cling to trying only things in which you can be perfect. Learning that excellent performance is not necessary, nor sufficient, for satisfaction will allow you to feel more relaxed. Possibly you can even try new things with a more relaxed attitude.

Another way to reduce your perfectionist self-talk is to substitute a more realistic self-talk. For instance, if you think, "I am not a good head nurse. I just can't manage this unit. I'm just not good enough," you will feel bad. You are overgeneralizing a mistake you have made to be symbolic of yourself as an incompetent person. A more realistic thought substitution would be, "That is not the best staff meeting I've run, but it was adequate." Negative, demanding mind chatter is almost a constant companion of a perfectionist. At least be specific in your criticism!

Writing down your irrational automatic thoughts may help trigger your sense of humor as you read your liturgy of absolutes. Writing them down puts you in the observer position. You know how ridiculous some of your actions were (as you look back) in the past. Well, this is looking back on your thoughts. Instead of allowing yourself to be consumed by self-critical or all-or-nothing thoughts, take the time to write them down.

Another key element is learning that people like you as much or more when you are not perfect. The only people who think less of you when you make a mistake are other perfectionists. I have found all perfectionists initially startled by finding that people do not reject them if they make a mistake or fail at something.

Assertiveness training techniques can help the perfectionist deal with the feared criticism. The perfectionist dreads criticism. The technique of *negative inquiry* is used to get a vague criticism to be specific. For example, the doctor says, "You are a stupid nurse." You could respond, "What did I do or say that made me look stupid?"

In a second assertiveness technique, *negative assertion,* you agree with the truth in the criticism. For instance, "you are always the last one to come and report off to me," is your charge nurse's criticism. The grain of truth in that statement is what you respond to, as you want to agree assertively with the negative statement. "You are right, I am the last person to report off today and yesterday; I am not always the last one," is an example of a negative assertion. Your critics will expect you to get defensive. When you do not, the emotional tone of the interaction tends to dampen. Both these techniques deal with the content of the criticism rather than your emotional response.

Fogging is another assertiveness technique. The technique is related to the concept of "fog." As you move into fog it does not resist you, you are able to push your way through easily. The fog also flows past you. In this technique the criticism is the fog you allow to flow past you. Consider the following example:

> *Patient:* "Nurses here don't spend enough time with patients."
> *Nurse:* "I can see why you would feel that way."
> *Patient:* "You, Nurse Hopkins, are unavailable to me."
> *Nurse:* (having spent most of morning in a meeting) "I understand you feel that way."

These fogging responses involve understanding the others' perception of a situation and show a nondefensive response.

These three assertiveness techniques, plus empathy, are important communication techniques to increase the satisfaction of interpersonal relationships. Being able to respond in some way other than defensively does a lot to improve a perfectionist's work and social relationships.

Empathy allows you to see the world through the critic's eye. Virginia Satir said this another way: "Communication is the greatest single factor affecting a person's health and their relationship to others."

Being able to manage criticism in a calm way is the dream of all perfectionists. Role rehearsal in assertiveness training or role playing in therapy will speed the process. Feeling okay, maintaining self-respect, and not getting defensive are all possible in the face of criticism.

A final message for perfectionists: Learn to make an average goal. Many of you are stymied by setting your perfect goals. Setting a goal to do something average can begin to teach you the joys that accompany nonperfection. I never believed satisfaction was possible, either, when I started to try this. If I had not learned this lesson, this book would have never been written. A perfect first draft is obviously a perfectionist desire.*

As a perfectionist, you compare yourself with some ideal image and rate yourself; the higher your score, the better you feel, because you are closer to perfect. You compare the postive and negative aspects about a particular trait in yourself and in others and decide whether you win or lose. Winning means you get to feel one-up or self-righteous; if you lose you feel inferior, resentful, or jealous. I personally do not care for the prizes you get for either winning or losing. There really is no winner in the comparison game.

TYPE A BEHAVIOR

Perfectionism and comparison are part of a pattern of behavior associated with coronary artery disease. Type A behavior is significantly correlated to individuals who have heart disease and have had coronary infarctions. Table 3-5 is a questionnaire to help you assess yourself on Type A behavior. For each question, choose one of the three following responses: always/usually; sometimes; seldom or never.

If your answers tend towards always/usually, then read the book by Friedman and Rosenman (1974). The statistics connecting Type A behavior with heart disease are very impressive. Ignoring your vulnerability to this health problem because you choose to see hypertension, high cholesterol, and smoking as more significant causes will only lead you to the sad conclusion that is being reached in heart disease studies.

Friedman (1981) reported that a study (Recurrent Coronary Preven-

---

*These ideas about how to deal with perfectionism come from three main sources: (1) my 33-year experience of dealing with perfectionism, (2) techniques I have taught my clients over the last 8 years, and (3) treatment approaches used at the University of Pennsylvania Mood Clinic (Burns, 1980).

Table 3-5
"HURRY SICKNESS" INDEX

1. Do you find yourself rushing your speech?
2. Do you hurry other people's speech by interrupting them with "umhm, umhm" or by completing their sentence for them?
3. Do you hate to wait in line?
4. Do you seem to be short of time to get everything done?
5. Do you detest wasting time?
6. Do you eat too fast?
7. Do you drive over the speed limit?
8. Do you try to do more than one thing at a time?
9. Do you become impatient if others do something too slowly?
10. Do you seem to have little time to relax and enjoy the time of day?
11. Do you find yourself overcommitted?
12. Do you jiggle your knees or tap your fingers?
13. Do you think about other things during conversations?
14. Do you walk fast?
15. Do you hate dawdling after a meal?
16. Do you become irritable if kept waiting?
17. Do you detest losing in sports or games?
18. Do you find yourself with clenched fists or tight neck or jaw muscles?
19. Does your concentration sometimes wander while you think about what is coming up later?
20. Are you a competitive person?

Reprinted from Schafer, W. *Stress, distress, and growth.* Davis, Calif.: Responsible Action, 1978. With permission.

tion Project) begun in 1979 involving 1,000 people has demonstrated a profoundly significant decrease in the incidence of heart disease in the group receiving Type A behavior modification compared to a control group. In the treatment group the incessant struggle against time and other persons (competition) that is seen in the Type A individual is reengineered through drills and group meetings. You can begin to reshape your Type A behavior by following the guidelines and exercises offered by Friedman and Rosenman (1974).

Ivancevich and Matteson (1980) conducted a descriptive survey using the Type A questionnaire to determine whether Type A nurses experience different stress than Type B nurses. The results showed that both saw responsibility for people and time pressures as significantly stressful. For Type A nurses politics and participation in decisions were most stressful, whereas for Type B nurses rewards and human resource development were seen as most stressful. Supervisors of nurses need to consider the difference in the needs of Type A and Type B nurses.

Ironically, driven, Type A people usually have not lost their sense of humor; however, they usually need help in perceiving their own ludicrous aspects, rather than relying on their repository of jokes and anecdotes.

USING HUMOR

Finding the humor in your antics with other people and their antics with you is my second trick in my "stress survival kit for life." The ability to laugh at yourself when you get caught in one of life's surprises—an unplanned happening that is out-of-your-control—will reduce your tension. Instead of standing there angry and screaming, or embarrassed and withdrawn, step back and take a look at the scene you are creating for the world to watch and enjoy the humor in your situation.

Humor comes in a variety of forms. The form of humor mentioned above is the humor of a funny story in its creation. You might as well enjoy the creation as well as the telling of it. How many times have you looked back and seen the humor in a situation that seemed awful when it occurred? Speed up your funny-bone reaction to replace the angry, jealous, or self-righteous reaction. Is not laughter a better experience than the three preceding feelings?

Laughter—the sounds that express joyousness and amusement—is a good stress reduction medicine. Norman Cousins (1979), in *Anatomy of an Illness*, relates how he used laughter as a cancer antidote. Being able to laugh at your problems helps prevent you from being overwhelmed by the weight of them.

DISCOUNTING AS AN INHIBITOR IN PROBLEM SOLVING

Sometimes it is important not to laugh problems away, but instead to confront them directly. Denying problems inhibits problem solving until the problem can no longer be ignored; often, by this time your stress level is high.

Problems—we all create them. I say "create" because no person's behavior and no environmental event is a problem until you define it as a problem. A little too existential? *Webster's* defines a *problem* as a "question proposed for solution or consideration." Each of you individually creates questions and then you seek answers. Obviously, what questions are proposed for solution is determined by the individual's needs. How can it be that the same situation is a problem for some and not for others?

Schiff (1975) speaks to the issue with an interesting slant. She states there are four levels of discounting (denying) that inhibit problem solving: The first level is discounting that a problem exists—literally denying the stimulus. At this level you will hear, "I didn't see blood on her dressing or hear her bell." "I didn't even notice the son was standing there watching until after the 'code' was over." "I did not see your request for the budget report by Tuesday." In all three examples the individual was unaware of the existence of a problem. Ignorance is bliss only in the short run.

The recognition of the stimulus begins the processing of information. If, however, you discount the significance or importance of the problem, then you are simply treating all incoming information the same. Recognizing the significance of the problem begins the processing at a second level. Missing the significance of an electrocardiogram tracing with sudden inverted T-waves or the significance of exhausted RNs doing double shifts could lead to hospital crisis and possibly patient death. Recognizing that there are significant problems motivates an individual to solve them.

Once you recognize the significance of the problem, you need to recognize the solvability of the problem. Denying the solvability of a problem is discounting on the third level; it leaves you feeling frustrated. Too often we hear, "Nursing has never been a profession and never will be." "Management has never supported nursing, why even try to talk with them." Denying the solvability of this professional issue, or the problem of unsupportive management just leads to a dead end.

The fourth level of discounting is denying your capacity to solve the problem. You recognize that you are gaining a significant amount of weight and that it is a solvable problem, but you feel that *you* cannot solve it. Other people may be able, but you are not able. Whether your reason is a sense of paralysis in seeing options or disappointment paralysis over failed choices, you experience an inability to solve this problem. The solution to recognizing your capacity involves recognizing your resources (encouragement, brainstorming, and expert resources.)

Problem solving is an important stress management skill. This skill is addressed in other ways in this book, such as the steps in problem solving (Chapter 7) and further identification of your problems (Chapter 8). Recognizing these levels of discounting is an initial step toward problem solving.

PERSONAL DEVELOPMENT

Increasing Self-Awareness

Solving problems is part of your personal development. Personal development involves keeping abreast of who you are and who you want to become. Your self-awareness is a key stress reducer.

Staying aware of yourself and your needs prevents destructive habits. Remember that nursing school instructor or that supervisor you swore you never wanted to be like? Remember how inflexible and opinionated he or she was, always needing to be right? Well, you could become like him or her if you fool yourself into total acceptance of the status quo. Do not overdose on security: security and stability need to be balanced with risk and change.

Along with creating your own change, you need to monitor your response to change. In order to have a less stressful life that incorporates change, your level of reactivity to change should allow you to feel that life is like riding a car over hilly country roads, not like riding the Sooper-Dooper-Looper roller coaster at Hershey Park. When life feels like a roller coaster or a bucking bronco you need help in reacting to change.

Calming your reactivity is achieved through seeing change as part of the total picture of a changing world. Seeing people's behaviors as designed to create uproar in your life borders on paranoia. People are just living their own lives. Taking their actions personally leads to anxiety and depression. According to your view, sometimes they are inconsiderate, incompetent, and irresponsible; many times their own view of their behavior is different. Your getting angry and upset hurts *you*. Your stress response of fighting or fleeing helps or hinders *you*.

Your level of reactivity also affects others. Someone does something you deem as inappropriate and you act angry, which then affects the rest of your staff. Some people give ulcers and some people get them! If you are an overreactor begin to take a look at how you respond to life situations. Is the situation or person that bad? Anger is not useful for solving problems, anger is an emotional release. The next time you encounter a situation that you usually overreact to, try to take the perspective of the other person involved. Furthermore, my grandmother was right—counting to ten helps.

Drama Triangle: Understanding and Preventing Interpersonal Conflict

Another way of looking at the issue of reactivity is by using the concept of the "drama triangle" developed by Karpman (1972), a transactional analysis therapist. The drama triangle explains, through the use of three main characters, the essence of overreactive scenes.

The three characters are Rescuer, Victim, and Persecutor. Both the Rescuer and the Persecutor believe that people are often not okay and in need of help, but they approach the issue differently. The Rescuer's stance is, "You are helpless and hopeless, let me help you." They are the helpers—overzealous, self-sacrificing, and often quietly auditioning for the most valued person. The difference between a helper and a Rescuer is that the Rescuer, when asked for help, does it all. Often the Rescuer does it without being asked, but looks a little resentful.

The Persecutor's stance is, "You are helpless and hopeless, but it is your own fault." The insinuation always is that if you were not so stupid, clumsy, or inept you would not need help. The Persecutor stance may feel less familiar to nurses than the Rescuer position, although all of you have on occasion taken this role.

The cry of the Victim is "I'm helpless and hopeless, help me, help me." This cry is not the cry of a person in grave danger and absolutely in need of help. People playing this role repeatedly need help in completing assignments, cannot seem to do their own problem solving, and whine whenever they complain.

The drama occurs when the players shift roles. You only need two, although three players can participate. For a real-life example let us take the case of Nurse Rescue, who has repeatedly stayed late to help Nurse Inept Victim to complete her patient assignment. One day Nurse Rescue cannot stay late. Nurse Victim cries out—just as your son or daughter does when you will not sew that Halloween costume or type that paper the night before it is due—"I thought I could count on you, just when I need you you are not there."

The shift in triangle roles has begun and so has the drama. Nurse Victim has now become the Persecutor. Guess what role Nurse Rescue has taken? Right, the role of the Victim with the wounded cry of, "After all I've done for her she treats me this way." This often is followed shortly by the move to Persecutor, with statements such as, "You are ungrateful. I've done a lot for you by staying late."

Having shifted around to complete the drama, the players may now recycle. I call guilt the "universal recycler," for having felt guilty the person begins to rescue again. Nurse Rescue's recycle line is, "I should have been more understanding of her. She is under a lot of stress." This guilt creates the process of overhelping once again.

One major rule of this game is that once you get on the triangle in any one of the three positions, you will have to switch to at least one other position before you can get off the triangle. Obviously, the idea is to avoid getting on the triangle. Notice the next time you end up as a Victim and see this concept in action.

Changing this pattern is like changing any other pattern. First, you must recognize that you are on the triangle: you recognize you have just made a mistake by rescuing. The second step is to be aware you are making a mistake *while* you are making it: you know you are playing Victim, but you just do not want to do the report; you know you could do it, but it is easier to let the other person rescue you. The third step is to

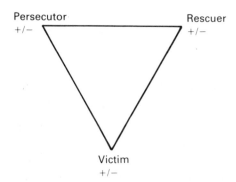

FIGURE 3-1. Drama triangle. [Adapted from Karpman, S. B. Fairy Tales and Script Drama Analysis. *Transactional Analysis Bulletin*, 1968, 7, 39–48.]

become aware *before* you step onto the triangle: stop yourself before you make the mistake. Changing the habit of rescuing others or persecuting others is just like changing any other habit: the change takes awareness, persistence, and patience.

Note the diagram in Figure 3-1 and remember a time you entered the drama triangle from the Rescuer position. Remember how you felt when the switch occurred and you felt like a Victim. Surely you want to avoid that feeling.

Getting Positive Recognition

When you get to the third step of the process described above, take time to give yourself recognition for your achievement. Getting recognition for your achievements is another stress preventer. Feeling that you are taken for granted and unappreciated by your spouse or your boss creates stress. Depression is always associated with the lack of positive recognition.

There are different varieties of positive recognition on two continuums: (1) verbal and nonverbal, and (2) conditional and unconditional. Verbal compliments are helpful in supporting nurses through long hours, as are nonverbal smiles, knowing nods, and even nurturing hugs. I always liked the bumper sticker, "Have you hugged a nurse today?" We sure could use more of those hugs!

The conditional and unconditional continuum involves rewards for "doing" and recognition for "being." "You did a good job of diabetic counseling with Mr. Smith," and "I appreciate your clear thinking in the emergency," are examples of conditional rewards that give the person credit for performance. The unconditional recognition is given just for your existence: for example, "I love you," or "I care about you." Many single nurses are starving for this type of recognition. Conditional recognition is important, however, I highly recommend building a suport group that feels comfortable giving unconditional verbal and nonverbal recognition.

Building Support Systems

The importance of a support system has been shown in many studies (Caplan, 1974; Pines & Aronson, 1981). The support of colleagues was found to be significant in reducing stress in several studies (Cassem & Hackett, 1975; Pines and Kafry, 1978; Pines & Maslach, 1978). Pines and Kafry (1978, p. 502) define *social support systems* as "Enduring interpersonal ties to a group of people who can be relied upon to provide feedback while sharing standards and values . . ." These support groups provide a protective buffer against work pressure. Pines and Kafry (1978, p. 502) note that "one of the most crucial elements in staff morale . . . is whether they had good working relationships with their colleagues." Supportive work groups, where responsibilities were shared, were experienced by professionals as less personally stressful.

Pines and Maslach (1978) recommend retreats for staff members as a way to build supportive work relationships. Katz (1978) states that mutual participation in the resolution of conflict and problems, as well as group members being respected as individuals and allowed to freely contribute their ideas for the betterment of the group, contributed to reducing work stress.

Support from others enriches the resources available on the job. A group of psychiatric clinical specialists formed a professional support group and found it useful in dealing with the frustration of multilevel demands for support, and productive as a source of stimulation (Johnson, Richardson, Von Endt, & Lindgren, 1982). Developing a professional support group is one way to reduce work stress. Kirschenbaum and Glaser (1978) and Marram (1973) offer ways to begin and maintain support groups.

Beyer and Marshall (1981) discuss the importance of the concept of collegiality among nurse educators; this includes confidence and trust, mutual help, mutual support, friendliness and enjoyment, team efforts toward goal achievement, creativity, open communication, and freedom from threat. They suggest programs dealing with conflict and sharing for the management of stress and burnout.

Cassem and Hackett (1975) describe group crisis meetings designed to foster a supportive environment in ICU units. There are four essential steps in the process:

1. The feelings must be identified and acknowledged.
2. Other members of the group must allow themselves to share, i.e., both empathize with the nurse who introduces the feeling and share their own perspective, even though it may be somewhat different.
3. It is necessary to examine, question the details, confess guilt where it is felt, give support, reinforcement, and praise where due.
4. Subsequent to these operations, the experience can be integrated and a proper perspective attained. (Cassem & Hackett, 1975, p. 255)

These concepts could be applied to other units within the hospital.

Discussion sessions for staff to ventilate feelings are also advocated by Eisendrath and Dunkel (1979), Huckabay and Jagla (1979), and Oskins (1979). ICU staff members need to get together with administrators for discussions of problems and solutions (Huckabay & Jagla, 1979). A nurse clinical specialist or liaison psychiatrist could act as a group facilitator, as well as a consultant for didactic talks and patient management.

At different times different means of support will need to be elicted. The types of support are divided into two categories: career and emotional. Career support could include a mentor, someone who will challenge you to achieve, to be creative—someone you respect in your field who you could learn from. Dr. Rodney Napier and Dr. Dorothy del Bueno are my challenging supports—name two for yourself.

Career support can also be given by someone who provides honest feedback on your work performance or just listens to your work problems. This nurse will affirm your ability as a nurse. Another source of comfort is a "bitch buddy"—someone who will listen to your catharsis and will not try initially to problem solve for you. This person knows, as a colleague, that the support you need is to have someone to listen. Name two people you have that fit the above descriptions. Unfortunately, many nurses fail to use this effective stress prevention mechanism because they do not fully understand its importance, its different functions, and how best to utilize it. In any work environment it is crucial to have someone who can provide technical support to actively listen without giving advice or making judgments (Pines & Aronson, 1981).

The second type of support is emotional. It is important to know that someone is in your corner, someone you can count on through thick and thin. If you win or lose does not matter to this person; this person is there by your side, although not necessarily in agreement. Who in your life provides this kind of support?

This support person may also act as what I call a "keeping me honest friend." We all can deny our responsibilities and rationalize our behavior. You need people who will support your personal growth by questioning your decisions and your efforts. If you actively use the defense mechanisms of denial and rationalization, this type of person can prove invaluable for you. List your two "keeping you honest friends."

Even though listening was mentioned before, it is important enough to mention again. Sharing your perception of reality with someone, knowing that person is listening, and then experiencing validation of your perception can be an effective stress preventer. You need people with whom you can share your downs and your ups—people who listen to your trivial everyday incidents, as well as your triumphs and your pains or frustration. These people add the dimension of sharing as part of a support system. Who are two people in your life who listen well to you and/or you can check out reality with?

If you had difficulty naming people who provide these types of support for you, take note that your support system is not solid. Some names may appear more than once, for these people fulfill several different support roles. At least five different names would provide you with a safe buffer.

A final word on support for those of you who have a hard time depending on others for anything. In order to care effectively for others, you need to get replenished. You are not a Florence Nightingale lamp ever-burning without new fuel. Delegating responsibilities at home and work, and allowing yourself the delicacy of dependence is a way of taking care of yourself while taking care of others.

Having a solid, stable support system is a key point in stress prevention, as is having a purpose for your life. A purpose in life provides direction for life's path. Without a purpose, life can feel aimless, out of control, or meaningless. You can use your support system to help guide you in achieving your purpose.

Developing a Life Purpose

Psychologists, philosophers, and spiritual teachers have taught us that having a purpose in life is important in creating a satisfying and fulfilling life. A satisfying and fulfilling life is a less stressful life.

Having a purpose toward which you direct your energies helps keep you focused on something more than the nitty-gritty negative occurrences you encounter daily. People without goals get aimlessly tossed about in their daily problems, whereas people with a purpose do not pay as much attention to these problems—they see them as a part of life, not life itself. Sometimes people confuse purpose and goals: goals are stepping stones to achieving your purpose.

Having a purpose in life involves focusing your attention on doing something that contributes to your fellow humans. Raising a child, developing an effective nursing management team, or providing the nursing

Table 3-6
COMFORT ZONE LIMITS

---

1. How many hours of sleep do you need?
2. How long can you work effectively before you need a break?
3. How long does your break need to be in order for you to be refreshed?
4. Do you know how you feel when you feel full, but not stuffed?
5. How many drinks can you have before you notice changes in yourself?
6. What are your signs of boredom (e.g., restlessness, confusion, spacing out)?
7. What are three requests you are likely to say "yes" to that tend to push you over the upper limit?
8. What limit do you repeatedly go over?

---

students with the best education possible are all examples of having a purpose in life. Contemplate your purpose. Having a purpose you can respect and feel proud of supports you in receiving the good will of others.

Knowing Your Comfort Zone

All these prevention ideas and skills need to be considered and learned to provide the necessary buffer for stress. Some of you can tolerate a larger degree of stress and still feel comfortable; others have a narrower range of tolerance. Whatever your limits, you need to consider stress prevention in the psychological realm.

We all have our limits. When you go over your limits your body breaks down with signs and symptoms of abuse, and your mind breaks down with overloaded circuits. Many times the reactions you see are due to this overload. The sooner you realize you are approaching your limits, the better able you will be to apply the brakes so that you do not come to a screeching halt. We all have a zone of comfort. When you go over the upper limit you feel overwhelmed—every request feels like a demand. When you go under the lower limit, you feel bored with your life.

Your comfort zone is the range of stimulation that is comfortable and healthy for you. Knowing what your limits are will help you stay within this zone. To know these limits better, answer the questions in Table 3-6. Preventing stress-related problems depends on your knowing and living within your comfort zone as much as you can.

In this chapter the focus has been on assessing your mind and emotional state. Gaining control over your emotions will greatly reduce your personal and work stress. In the next chapter the focus is on identifying and changing addictive patterns.

4

Behavioral Strategies: Recognizing and Changing Your Addictions

THE EXTENT OF THE PROBLEM

There are dozens of ways to cope with stress. One of the chief short-term coping methods people use to decrease their tension is drugs. Drugs are used to dampen the psychological symptoms of anxiety and depression. Physical symptoms are also treated with drugs. Sleeping pills to treat insomnia, Valium to relax muscle tension, and coffee to treat fatigue are just a few examples of drug use.

Some drugs people use are available only with a prescription, some are sold over the counter, and some are illegal. Since the illegal ones are the strongest drugs, the people who use them are usually in the most serious trouble. Using illegal drugs to cope with life's ups and downs is a sure sign you are failing to cope with your stress and you are in trouble. The trouble is increased by the social implications of using these drugs, the physical damage they cause to the body, and the possible permanent psychological changes they can generate.

Using prescription drugs is often the upper middle-class way of handling stress. Valium, Librium, Percodan, sleeping pills, and diet pills—all are used to cope with the tensions of career and family. The ever increasing financial pressure and achievement focus take their toll on people who are not managing their stress well. Drugs of this type can be used to help slow the mind or lose the unsightly fat; however, the psychological addiction and sometimes physical addiction is a high price to pay for stress reduction.

The mildest form of drugs is the over the counter variety. Caffeine-laced cold preparations, coffee, tea, cola, chocolate, and alcohol are used to quiet the nerves. Add refined foods, cigarettes, and sugar, and you have the middle-class equivalent of the drug culture.

Sometimes people are not aware that they are using drugs to cope with stress. Using the drug has become a habit. You may have used this substance for so long you may not even know you are addicted—the drug has become a part of your everyday life. Whether it is speed, diet pills, or caffeine, you look forward to the drug; it helps you get through the day, and the vague guilt you feel for taking the drug fades when it begins to take effect.

How extensive is the problem of addiction in nurses? It is estimated that there are 40,000 alcoholic nurses in the United States (Bissell, 1979). This represents 1 to 2 percent of the practicing nurses. The rate of narcotics addiction among nurses closely parallels that among physicians—their rate is 30 to 100 times greater than in the general population (Murray, 1974). The population equivalent of ten nursing schools and three medical schools is lost each year to narcotics addiction (Garb, 1965).

This problem of addiction is being addressed on a national and on some state levels. The American Nurses Association (ANA), in 1982, created a Nursing Task Force on Addiction and Psychological Disturbances. Its task was "to formulate guidelines that state nurses' associations can use for developing programs to help nurses whose practice is impaired by alcoholism, drug abuse, or psychological dysfunctions" ("Help for the Helper," 1982).

Georgia, Maryland, Ohio, and Tennessee have active programs, and three other states have, as of the beginning of 1982, committees actively working to develop programs. Maryland's program began in 1980, and in the first 18 months it had contact with 57 nurses. The Ohio program found that very few calls come from nurses seeking help; most have been referred by colleagues, friends, or family. In Georgia, more nurses were coming to the program than the volunteer nurses could handle. The program has been expanded with the help of the Georgia Nurses Association ("What the SNA's Are Doing," 1982).

In this chapter the focus is on you truly learning if the use of drugs is a problem for you. Treatment strategies to deal with the problem are offered, and by the end of this chapter you will have gained at least the beginning of the information necessary to deal with your use of drugs. If you find you have no problem, then perhaps you can think of someone who needs to read this chapter, and give it to that person. You could help someone begin the first stage of treatment—recognition of the problem.

For instance, almost all people who smoke know that they should stop. What are effective ways to bring a person to the decision to quit? This motivation to quit, once activated, is so powerful that a three-pack-a-day smoker can quit and never return to smoking. What motivation could possibly bring people to give up a long-term, daily, reinforced habit that they enjoy?

The answer lies in understanding that what looks like a large, sudden change is a gradually evolving process. It is likely that the person has been collecting and processing information leading to that decision long before the decision is acted upon. To help you make the decision to quit your addiction, the consequences of these addictive actions are pointed out and guidelines for changing these behaviors are presented. These discussions will help you gain the information necessary to trigger the change process. In making any change, you give up something and you gain something. The dynamics and difficulties of changing addictive behaviors, the triggering keys, and specific suggestions on how to change are discussed. Individual addictions are focused upon, along with their diagnostic signs and symptoms, treatment, and prevention strategies. (The process for using this information is delineated in Chapter 8.)

All the desire to change will not change a habit if the desire is based on unrealistic and unmanageable guidelines. The guidelines help support you down the rocky road of change. Understanding some of the dynamics of addictive behavior will help you begin to comprehend the difficulty people encounter in giving up addictions.

DYNAMICS AND DIFFICULTIES IN CHANGING ADDICTIONS

Of all the psychological, pharmacological, and sociological theories to explain addiction, only the pharmacological remains constant. Our understanding of the physical process the body undergoes, the behavioral signs, and the predictability of the effects has not changed. Personality theories have been discarded and new ideas about the origin of addictive processes are emerging. Psychiatric diagnoses have not appeared to be helpful in determining the course of treatment for addictions in study after study. As Nyswander remarked in 1959, "We must conclude that addiction may exist in individuals with almost any psychic organization, and that they may overcome the illness without necessarily undergoing any obvious changes in the personality" (p. 618). Unfortunately, we are still not sure of the psychodynamics involved in addictions. Differing opinions exist, and therefore only an overall view is presented here.

Nurses often do not see alcoholism as a disease. They remember learning in nursing school that it is a symptom of an underlying problem. This only confirms their worst fears—that if they stopped drinking an underlying, more severe problem would surface. The truth is that the usual underlying problem is simply low self-esteem. This problem can be covered up by high achievement and outward gaiety: one nurse recalled that her worst years were her most successful professionally. As the disparity between how she presented herself to the world and how she felt increased, so did her drinking.

Some authors examine personality traits and dynamics. This overall picture must include a focus on the emotional, cognitive, and behavioral aspects of the addiction. At present, the premorbid personality pattern is not clear. However, some characteristics repeatedly seen in studies (Belfer, Shader, Carroll, & Harmaty, 1971; Jones, 1971; Kinsey, 1966; Lindbeck, 1972; Wikler, 1953) suggest some specific dynamics. Basically, the person is not able to fulfill the need for an intimate relationship or the need to express self in an aggressive way. The anxiety and stress created by not meeting these needs is overwhelming and the individual seeks the drug to alleviate the anxiety. The alcoholic chooses a drug to release inhibitions to become exhibitionistic. Tranquil and now feeling in control, the Valium and marijuana user fits perfectly the British definition of an addict—a person who feels normal on drugs (Nyswander, 1959, p. 616).

Understanding the emotional life of a person with addictive behaviors is essential in establishing effective change guidelines. Some drug users feel unable to control their emotions, so they choose substances that dull their emotions. Others have surpressed their emotions so much that depression, loneliness, emptiness, boredom, and despair lead them to use amphetamines and caffeine for stimulation.

A few studies have been done on addicted nurses. Bissell's (1979) study of 100 alcoholic nurses revealed some interesting personality statistics on nurses. Most of these nurses were at the top of their class, held advanced degrees, held demanding and responsible jobs, were highly respected in their jobs, and were ambitious and achievement oriented. This is hardly the image you have of the stereotypical alcoholic. A major study of 90 female addicts (Poplar, 1969) showed that they began "using drugs legitimately as a form of self-medication for physical or emotional, personal or job-related problems" (Jefferson & Ensor, 1982). They were using drugs to cope with their stress. The study also showed that they tended to use the drugs in private to protect their reputation. Again, this does not support the image of the "gang hanging out together doing drugs."

Drugs and alcohol are used to manage the mental and emotional consequences of stress. Depression and anxiety are the two most common psychiatric diagnoses. Using assorted drugs to mask these difficulties is not solving your stress problem. You actually are exacerbating the problem because the real problem remains untreated. You need to realize that you are using certain behaviors to cope that will actually make matters worse.

These behaviors are difficult to change because they do relieve psychic and physical pain that stress creates, and you try to fool yourself into believing the cause is gone. You may rationalize that you are using the alcohol to adjust to a new job, but you may be drinking more in an effort to get the same effect. Dealing with the cause of the anxiety or depression relieves the need for a drugged emotional life.

The likelihood of being able to change is directly related to the motivation to change. "He who is forced against his will is of his own opinion still" clearly states the importance of motivation. In order to stimulate the motivation to change, it is important to understand the emotional life of a person involved in addictive behaviors.

The first step toward changing addictive behaviors is knowing the facts. One fact many people forget in their times of self-depreciation is that the change is difficult. For perfectionists, the path of changing an addictive behavior is paved with failures. Most people have multiple regressions during the process; how you view your regression is very important. Your view of your regression may be influenced by unrealistic expectations. This is one reason it is recommended to be part of a group. The support for change and confrontation of unrealistic expectations is a great help.

It is very important to remember that unrealistic, unmanageable change goals are frequently the cause of failure. Creating success experiences by expecting and completing small changes is the key, because seeing yourself as a success makes changing easier than seeing yourself as a failure. Therefore, any change program involves many small goals that you strive toward and successfully achieve. In order to climb a tree you need to reach for a branch that is realistic for you to reach, otherwise you will fall out of the tree into failure! Success in completing small changes supports major changes.

Even with the step-by-step change process, trying to make too many changes at once creates failure. Change shakes up the balance of a person. The individual has difficulty feeling centered. The body and mind go into shock with too many changes, and the individual seeks stability through old habits. In other words, tackling too many changes at once will actually increase your chance of failing. Methods to use to support changes in your life are given in some detail throughout this book. I suggest you postpone deciding which change you want to tackle until you have finished reading the whole book.

Changing is also difficult for some people because an underlying depression leads to basic attitudes of sadness and futility. Change is impossible if the individual sees the attempt to as futile and insignificant.

The sense of futility is often the result of repeated failures at unrealistic and unplanned for changes. Giving up an addiction involves taking on something else. The information in this chapter will help you devise a plan to lose an addiction and gain freedom from dependence on drugs.

Addictive substances are dysfunctional stress relievers. For example, all nurses in a New York City study (Jaffe, 1982) stated that stress was one of the conditions under which they drank. Drugs actually create more havoc with the body's biological stress response mechanism. *These substances exacerbate stress.* Some of these substances overstimulate the body and others alter the natural body functioning by dulling the warning signal of pain. Bodily signs and symptoms, as well as signs of abuse, all point to the need for you to develop more effective behavioral methods to reduce stress.

SUBSTANCES OF ABUSE
LEADING TO ADDICTIVE COPING

In Table 4-1 the drugs that are discussed in this section are listed. Begin your assessment by noting the answer that most closely approximates the amount of drug you use on a daily average. (In this inventory sugar is considered a drug.)

Add up the number of points you have and see below for the interpretation of your score:

0–6 points. If your score is based primarily on one substance, then you are quite likely to be using that drug to cope. If your points are scattered across a number of items, however, it is more likely that you are a victim of your own poor health habits.

7–11 points. Your score indicates that you may be using drugs to cope. You probably will deny or discount that drugs are a problem for you; however, my recommendation is that you take heed of your score. If you think you do not have an addiction to any one of the substances, try doing without the substances on which you checked 3–4 for 2 weeks and see how you feel. Your body and mind will tell you. (Check with a doctor for an appropriate withdrawal schedule, especially for barbiturates and amphetamines.)

12 or more points. You are abusing drugs in order to cope with psychological pain. You may firmly believe it is all physical pain, but the mind is always connected with body pain. The pain could be decreased

Table 4-1
DRUG ABUSE INVENTORY

		Points			
Substance	Amount[†]	0.5	1	2	3
Alcohol (including wine/beer)	Drinks	3–5/wk	1–2	3–4	5+
Tranquilizers	Times	occ.[*]	1	2–3	4+
Pain Medications	Times	occ.	1	2–3	4+
Sleeping pills		1–2/mo	1/wk	2–3/wk	every night
Cigarettes	Packs	occ.	$\frac{1}{2}$	$1-1\frac{1}{2}$	2+
Marijuana	Joints	occ.	2–3/wk	1–2	3+
Amphetamines	Pills	occ.	2–3/wk	1–2	3+
Coffee/tea/cola	Cups	occ.	1–2	3–4	5+
Sugar treats	Items containing sugar	1–3/wk	1–2	3–4	5+

*Occ.: occasionally.
†Amount per day, unless otherwise noted.

with some of the methods mentioned in this chapter and in Chapter 2. Drugs are only one way to cope with pain, there are other ways to cope with your stress.

With the information you learned about your potential addictive actions, please begin reading the following sections with the intention of finding the motivation to give up your addiction. You can find other ways to cope effectively with your anxiety and stress; many are offered in this book.

Dealing with Alcohol

The questionnaire presented in Table 4-2 is used by Alcoholics Anonymous. Answer this questionnaire to help yourself asess whether or not drinking is a problem in your life. The questions will help you learn which behaviors are correlated with problem drinking.

If you have answered "yes" to three or more of these test questions, you would be considered an alcoholic by Alcoholics Anonymous. An alcoholic is someone who is to some degree out of control of his or her drinking. Obviously, the "street people" have a lower degree of control than the nurses who increasingly are getting drunk at parties and work with hangovers. Too often, these hangovers are brushed aside by the nurses, their colleagues, and their supervisors as unimportant.

Table 4-2
ALCOHOL ABUSE QUESTIONNAIRE

1. Do you require a drink the next morning?
2. Do you prefer to drink alone?
3. Is your drinking harming your family in any way?
4. Do you lose time from work due to drinking?
5. Do you crave a drink at a definite time daily?
6. Do you get the shakes unless you continue drinking?
7. Has drinking made you irritable?
8. Does drinking make you careless of your family's welfare?
9. Have you harmed your husband or wife since drinking?
10. Has drinking changed your personality?
11. Has drinking caused you bodily complaints?
12. Does drinking make your restless?
13. Does drinking cause you to have difficulty sleeping?
14. Has drinking made you more impulsive?
15. Have you less self-control since drinking?
16. Has your initiative decreased since drinking?
17. Has your ambition decreased since drinking?
18. Do you lack perseverance in pursuing a goal since drinking?
19. Do you drink to obtain social ease?
20. Do you drink for self-encouragement?
21. Do you drink to relieve marked feelings of inadequacy?
22. Has your sexual potency suffered since drinking?
23. Has jealousy in general increased since drinking?
24. Do you show marked dislikes and hatreds since drinking?
25. Do you show marked moodiness as a result of drinking?
26. Has your drinking made you more sensitive?
27. Are you harder to get along with since drinking?
28. Do you turn to an inferior environment since drinking?
29. Is drinking endangering your health?
30. Is drinking endangering your peace of mind?
31. Is drinking making your home life unhappy?
32. Is drinking jeopardizing your business?
33. Is drinking clouding your reputation?
34. Is drinking disturbing the harmony of your life?
35. Has your efficiency decreased since drinking?
36. Have you ever had a complete loss of memory while, or after, drinking?
37. Have you ever felt, when or after drinking, an inability to concentrate?
38. Have you ever felt remorse after drinking?
39. Has a physician ever treated you for drinking?
40. Have you ever been hospitalized for drinking?

The effects of overdrinking are usually first felt in family relationships. Because alcoholics are harder to get along with, their home life becomes unhappy. Alcoholics become careless about the welfare of their families, sometimes even to the degree of committing child or mate abuse. Their work is also affected at some point because of lost time, lax producitivity, or difficulty in getting along with people. Sometimes it is not until they are in jeopardy of losing their jobs that alcoholics admit that drinking is a problem.

The effects of alcohol on the mind and the body create physiological changes that endanger physical and emotional health. Alcohol as a drug acts as a depressant, but it initially stimulates the nervous system, creating a feeling of elation. This drug-created high enables the alcoholic to take risks by acting impulsively. The exhibitionistic behaviors of an alcoholic are actually a result of this freeing of control. The loss of control varies in intensity; sometimes it is quieter in appearance. This individual shows decreased initiative and efficiency, a lack of perserverance, and continuing withdrawal from the social mainstream. The drunk sitting all alone, glass in hand, looking remorseful is an accurate picture of many alcoholics.

Long before they reach that point, however, there are many instances of overdrinking and denial. Other signs you may recognize in yourself or another include increasing jealousy, feeling slighted easily, and markedly disliking others. These personality changes are often gradual, as is the development of sexual impotency. The effects of the drug lead to a loss of control over the body and the mind. The inability to concentrate and a loss of memory during or after drinking are often joked-about signs of alcoholism. Not everyone who drinks has these signs; there are physiological reasons for these signs occurring in the body of an alcoholic.

Some of the changes that you could notice in yourself or a colleague are listed in Table 4.3. This is also a list of the changes that a nursing supervisor needs to document.

Your identification with some of these signs and symptoms may have surprised you. Do yourself a favor and do not lapse back into denial. You can deal with the anxiety of knowing you are an alcoholic. With support, you can stop letting overdrinking hurt your life and find other ways to control your stress.

Alcoholism is often not diagnosed until the person no longer can deal with life and alcohol at the same time. It is estimated that currently about nine million people in the United States habitually abuse alcohol to such a degree that they constitute a major problem to themselves and to the public as a whole. Only five percent of these are skid row derelicts. One-half of the alcoholic individuals in the nation are employed (Deluca, 1981).

Alcoholism is often an accepted social behavior, just as gluttony is at parties. There are no figures on alcoholism among nurses in comparison

Table 4-3
SIGNS AND SYMPTOMS OF THE ALCOHOLIC NURSE

1. More irritable with patients and colleagues; withdrawn; mood swings
2. Isolated; wants to work night shifts; lunches alone; avoids informal staff get-togethers
3. Elaborate excuses for behavior such as being late for work
4. Blackouts: complete memory loss for events, conversations, phone calls to colleagues; euphoric recall of events on the floor
5. Job shrinkage: does minimal work necessary
6. Difficulty meeting schedules and deadlines
7. Illogical or sloppy charting
8. Increasingly absent from duty with inadequate explanations; long lunch hours; sick leave after days off
9. Calls in to request compensatory time at the beginning of shift

Reprinted from *List of 9 signs and symptoms of the alcoholic nurse*. Columbus, Ohio: Ohio Nurses Association Peer Assistance Program for Nurses, 1981. With permission.

to the general population. What is your guess? Your guess will have to incorporate some people you may have not initially thought of prior to considering Tables 4-2 and 4-3.

Whether you are surprised, depressed, scared, or confirmed, do not pass Tables 4-2 and 4-3 off as nonsense quizzes. Just sit for a minute and let yourself contemplate, "Now what?" The hardest phrase you will ever utter is "I am an alcoholic." Remember, however, that only after you utter it are you on the road to recovery.

HELPING THE ALCOHOLIC NURSE

Some people have quit abusing alcohol without the help of profes-sionals and Alcoholics Anonymous. These people, who luckily either caught the disease early enough or were able to pull themselves up by their bootstraps, are rare alcoholics. Some people who use alcohol to cope with stress are not alcoholic; however, if they continue to use alco-hol as a stress and anxiety reliever they are likely to get hooked into drinking for social ease and/or drinking to relieve painful feelings of inadequacy, inferiority, and guilt.

You will soon know if you can control your drinking to a safe level. All you need to do is to set a goal to reduce your drinking, for instance, from four drinks to one drink. If you can meet your goal consistently and continually, then you probably need not worry about alcoholism. How-ever, if you set the goal and do not meet it, you should seek the help of a counselor. Playing with a drinking problem is like playing with fire: the burns often leave permanent scars. Jefferson and Ensor (1982) list a num-ber of "do's and don'ts" for intervention strategies for colleagues and supervisors of alcoholic and drug-addicted nurses. They cover interventions for the acutely intoxicated nurse, the nonacute problem, and the posttreatment phase. They emphasize that the only choice that is clearly wrong is to do nothing.

Jaffe (1982) studied 10 nurses who participated in Alcoholics Anonymous; five of the ten also sought the additional assistance of psychotherapy. Alcoholics Anaonymous still has the best track record in helping people with alcoholism.*

Alcoholics Anonymous is an organization designed to provide you with the tools to overcome your drinking problem. It was founded in 1935 by a New York stockbroker and an Ohio surgeon who had been hopeless drunks. More and more people began to hear about it, and soon many alcoholics found they did not have to let their illness do that much damage. The number of Alcoholics Anonymous groups has grown to 40,000 local groups in 110 counties; total membership is estimated to be over 1 million. Organizations to help the families (spouses and children) of alcoholics were started several years later; they are called Alanon and Alateen.

Through the example and friendship of the recovered alcoholics in Alcoholics Anonymous, new members are encouraged to stay away from drinking "one day at a time." By keeping alcohol out of their systems, they give their bodies a chance to get well. They begin to straighten out their drinking by following "12 Steps" to recovery. These steps provide guidelines for the alcoholic to live a happier and more useful life.

Alcoholics Anonymous does several things for the treatment of the individual that need further elaboration. You do not need to be an alcoholic to be an effective helper; but it sure helps. The cons people use on themselves and others to maintain a behavior are more readily detected when you have used them yourself.

Availability to each other as support 24 hours a day, the buddy system, frequently meeting and sharing with each other, and the availability of important information all add up to giving members the experience of "you are there when I need you." These techniques are useful for people suffering with alcoholism as well as other addictions. They learn that they do not have to continue to believe that they are weak or that they should never ask for help. They learn to trust people and realize that the feeling of loneliness should not be treated with alcohol.

There are other approaches to dealing with alcoholism besides the psychological approaches of Alcoholics Anonymous and counseling programs. All of them, however, require abstinence from alcohol. In nutritional programs the focus is on the faulty carbohydrate metabolism of the

---

*For information on your local chapters call or write Alcoholics Anonymous World Services, Inc., Box 459, Grand Central Station, New York, NY 10163, (212) 686-1100.

individual, as well as a possible allergy to alcohol. Some studies have demonstrated nutritional and metabolic difficulties that result from the abuse of alcohol (Burch & Ansari, 1968; Gordon & Southren, 1977). However, the excessive ingestion of alcohol is more often seen as the cause, not the consequence of poor diet. Alcohol taken in small doses does not have a toxic effect. Large doses of alcohol are very toxic to the finely tuned metabolic system. Since alcoholics frequently substitute other drugs for alcohol, it is apparent that their craving is for the *effect* of alcohol. Any treatment program has to deal with all the ramifications of that need in order to succeed.

PREVENTION: FINDING AN ALTERNATIVE STRESS RELIEVER

If, in fact, the craving is for the effects of alcohol, then prevention strategies need to be centered around finding natural ways to alleviate anxiety and stress and induce a sense of well-being. (See the section titled Antiaddiction Approaches, page 98.)

The prevention of alcoholism needs to begin early in the educational system to create a shift in attitude toward drinking. At present, alcohol is seen as a sanctioned means to relieve stress. Only after a drinker becomes a social hazard is drinking considered a problem.

Because early indicators of problem drinking are ignored, most alcoholic nurses are experiencing real problems before they take seriously the possibility of alcoholism (Isler, 1978). The best way to prevent alcoholism is to find alternative ways to raise your self-esteem so that you can be the outgoing, assertive, tension-free person you desire to be.

Dealing with Drugs

Drug misuse is a growing national problem. As more drugs become marketable, the illegal trade in these drugs creates multiple law enforcement problems. Drugs prescribed for the treatment of physical and emotional illnesses are being abused by individuals seeking relief from the depression and anxiety caused by an overload of stress. Coping with stress by using drugs can lead down the same dead-end path as using alcohol.

A significant factor contributing to the use of drugs by nurses is their easy access to pills, narcotics, and prescriptions. A typical case would be Ruth, who began taking Librax for repeated gastric problems. She noticed that she felt she could cope with the stress of her ICU job more easily. Later she had dental work done and was given a prescription for Percodan. This yellow tablet was a constant companion of hers for two years. She feigned other illnesses in order to receive the drug. She began to forge prescriptions and steal from the unit. Ruth even went as far as taking patient's medications. She did not see herself as addicted. Fortunately a nurse supervisor did, and after one month of being drug-free in a therapeutic community and one year of psychotherapy, Ruth is doing well.

"A drug is a substance that has an effect upon the body or mind" (National Clearing House for Drug Abuse Information, 1981). Drug dependence is a state of psychological or physical dependence, or both, which results from chronic, periodic, or continuous use. Not everyone who uses mind-altering chemicals becomes dependent on them. Habituation is the psychological desire to repeat the use of the drug for emotional reasons. The escape from stress and tension by the dulling of reality and euphoria is one reason drugs come to be used habitually. Although reports indicate a high rate of drug use in our society, many people who use drugs do not become habitual users and even fewer become addicted.

Addiction is a physical dependence upon a drug. The development of tolerance and withdrawal signs are considered part of the criteria for defining an addiction. Larger and larger amounts of the drug are needed to produce the same effect. The withdrawal signs are avoided as one uses the addicting drug repeatedly to deal with life's problems.

Every drug is harmful if taken in excess. The fact that certain drugs can produce beneficial results has produced the false notion that pills can solve all problems. Many drugs temporarily allow their users to evade frustrations, to lessen depression and feelings of alienation, or to escape from themselves. This flight from the problem does not allow the individual to develop effective stress treatment and preventive coping patterns.

Two different types of drugs can become addictive: those that create an elated feeling and those that create a calm feeling. Both allow the individual to experience relief from the pain of inner conflict and escape to a temporary reality. The drugs that have a calming effect, such as tranquilizers, pain medications, and sleeping pills are discussed here; those that elate are considered in the section Dealing with Stimulants.

Signs of drug addiction need to be confronted, for a nurse addicted to drugs is dangerous to him- or herself, and to patients. Take note if the signs and symptoms in Table 4-4 apply to you; if not, then do they apply to a colleague?*

TRANQUILIZERS, SLEEPING PILLS,
AND PAIN MEDICATIONS

One-half of the prescription drugs sold in the United States are Valium and Librium. Valium is not only the most widely prescribed tranquilizer in the world, it is the most frequently prescribed medication of any

---

*For information and help you can contact World Services Office of Narcotics Anonymous, P.O. Box 622, Sun valley, CA 91352, (213) 768–6203.

Table 4-4
SIGNS AND SYMPTOMS OF THE DRUG-ADDICTED
NURSE

1. Extreme and rapid mood swings: irritable with patients, then calm after taking drugs
2. Wears long sleeves all the time
3. Suspicious behavior concerning controlled drugs
   a. Consistently signs out more controlled drugs than anyone else
   b. Frequently breaks or spills drugs
   c. Purposely waits until alone to open narcotics cabinet
   d. Consistently volunteers to be Med Nurse
   e. Disappears into bathroom directly after being in narcotics cabinet.
   f. Vials appear altered
   g. Incorrect narcotic count
   h. Discrepancies between reports by the nurse's patients and other patients on effective medications, etc
   i. Patient complains that pain medications dispensed by this nurse are ineffective
   j. Defensive when questioned about medical errors
4. Too many medication errors
5. Too many controlled drugs broken or spilled
6. Illogical or sloppy charting
7. Frequently absent from unit
8. Comes to work early and stays late for no reason—hangs around
9. Uses sick leave lavishly

Reprinted from *List of 9 signs and symptoms of drug addicted nurse.* Columbus, Ohio: Ohio Nurses Association Peer Assistance Program for Nurses, 1981. With permission.

kind. In less than three decades these pills have come to account for an estimated 40 percent of the reported $40 billion in annual drug sales by Hoffman-La Roche pharmaceutical house. In 1978, 2.3 billion tablets of Valium were sold (Colen, 1980).

Valium is safe and nonaddictive if taken for a short period of time. Studies have shown, however, that a person who takes as little as two to three times the recommended maximum daily dose of Valium can get hooked. For most addicts, Valium is like a psychic aspirin, taken to ease life's pains. The danger of Valium, like other addictive drugs, is that it works in relieving stress. People need to learn ways to deal with stress other than blotting it out with drugs. Blunting symptoms of stress, in the long run, creates additional health problems.

Sleeping pills, pain medication, and other drugs with tranquilizing properties put you in a fog similar to the fog of drunkeness. Drugs and alcohol sooth tension and anxiety. Their numbing effects prevent you from recognizing that pain and anxiety are the body's signs that something is wrong. Instead of saying "my mind is warning me," people seek to shut down the warning system.

These drugs are often discounted as not creating a significant problem. They are probably the drugs most abused by nurses. Until 1975 Valium and Librium were free in most patient medication drawers. Today they are regulated because of gross abuse. If you believe you are not addicted, and you choose to give up these drugs and try natural means to cope with life, please beware. Here is a list of withdrawal signs to be alert to:

Craving	Shivers
Irritability	Gastrointestinal disturbances
Depression	Loss of appetite
Anxiety	Hot flashes
Aching	Sleepiness, drowsiness
Nervousness, restlessness	Insomnia
Headache	Difficulty in concentrating

For the nurses I have treated, Percodan and barbituate withdrawal was very uncomfortable. With some substances it is very dangerous to withdraw suddenly. Check with a physician and develop a withdrawal treatment program. Do begin to consider the possibility of giving up these drugs. Perhaps you are free of this drug problem and could spend your energy helping someone else through confrontation or caring support.

TREATMENT PROGRAMS

Drug addiction treatment varies from terrible to refreshing. Your economic status, the drug you are addicted to, and your ability to quit "cold turkey" determine where you get treatment. The process is difficult, but never as difficult as you anticipated once you get to the other side. For most people coping with stress is possible without drugs.

How can you tell a good place of treatment? The following is a list compiled by talking with drug counselors and drug users:

- Some employees are ex-drug users.
- Group psychotherapy is part of the process.
- Individuals are caringly confronted on their behavior.
- There is supportive milieu.
- Stress management is addressed as an issue.

You may think that drugs are not a problem for you or other nurses in your hospital. You, as a nurse manager, may suspect that some of your staff is abusing, or, as a nurse instructor, you may suspect a student. Their admitting their addiction is no easier than you admitting yours.

The Georgia Nurses Association Impaired Nurse Program assists nurses in a three-pronged program: (1) education to spread the word, (2) entry into treatment to begin the recovery process, and (3) rehabilitation to return the nurse to productive practice ("What the SNA's Are Doing," 1982). Programs such as these are needed in all states so that nurses can stop the addiction process and learn other methods to cope with stress.

A note on sleeping medications: most sleeping medications set up a vicious cycle of sleep disturbance that feeds on the need for relaxation. Sleep is a time to relax. If you cannot sleep, that means you are not relaxed; put the relaxation exercise (page 21) on tape and play it at bedtime to help you relax enough to fall asleep.

Dealing with Cigarettes

The nicotine in the cigarettes you smoke is a drug, and—as those who have abruptly quit smoking can attest—there are withdrawal signs when you stop using this drug. In fact, in 1980 the American Psychiatric Association listed tobacco dependence in the *Diagnostic and Statistical Manual of Mental Disorders;* it is said to exist if the individual is unable to quit (or cut down) even in the face of obvious physical complications.

Most people are not aware that they take cigarettes when stressed; the connection between the stress and the taking of a cigarette has become automatic. The cigarette serves as a stimulant. As a nurse, you know that you rarely treat stress with stimulants. Quitting smoking can be a stressful experience in itself; however, in the long run you will experience less stress without cigarettes.

A nurse once told me her story of quitting. The first time she quit was after she saw an autopsy of one of her favorite patients who had died of lung cancer. He reminded her of her father (her father died of cancer). She quit on the spot. Two years later, when she and her husband separated, she started smoking again. Five years later, when she totaled her car and had to lie in a hospital bed, she was glad she was alive and quit smoking again. She has remained off cigarettes 6 years.

The impetus to stop has to be very strong. I think that the only reason people quit is that they believe if they do not quit they will die of cancer or some other disease related to smoking, such as heart disease. For some people, the connection between smoking and fatal disease takes longer to register; others comprehend the connection more quickly. What would it take for you to stop?

Please give various reasons for smoking. In Table 4-5 are some statements made by people to describe what they get out of smoking cigarettes. How often do you feel this way when smoking?

Smokers, take time to think about what your prime reasons for

Table 4-5
WHY DO YOU SMOKE?

Assign one number to each question, according to the following scale:

1 = Never

2 = Seldom

3 = Occasionally

4 = Frequently

5 = Always

Note that it is important to answer *every* question.

A. I smoke cigarettes in order to keep myself from slowing down.
B. Handling a cigarette is part of the enjoyment of smoking it.
C. Smoking cigarettes is pleasing and relaxing.
D. I light up a cigarette when I feel angry about something.
E. When I have run out of cigarettes I find it almost unbearable until I can get them.
F. I smoke cigarettes automatically without even being aware of it.
G. I smoke cigarettes to stimulate myself, to perk myself up.
H. Part of the enjoyment of smoking a cigarette comes from the steps I take to light up.
I. I find cigarettes pleasurable.
J. When I feel uncomfortable or upset about something, I light up a cigarette.
K. When I am not smoking a cigarette I am very much aware of the fact.
L. I light up a cigarette without realizing I still have one burning in the ashtray.
M. I smoke cigarettes to give myself a "lift."
N. When I smoke a cigarette, part of the enjoyment is watching the smoke as I exhale it.
O. I want a cigarette most when I am comfortable and relaxed.
P. When I feel "blue" or want to take my mind off cares and worries, I smoke cigarettes.
Q. I get a real gnawing hunger for a cigarette when I haven't smoked for a while.
R. I've found a cigarette in my mouth and didn't remember putting it there.

How to score

Tally the numbers you have chosen for the above questions as shown in the "equations" below. For example, taking the first equation (A + G + M = Stimulation), substitute the number you have chosen in answer to question A for the "A" in the equation, to question G for the "G," and to question M for the "M." Add these three scores to get your total for "Stimulation."

Scores can vary from 3 to 15. Any score of 11 and above is high; any score of 7 and below is low.

A + G + M = Stimulation
B + H + N = Handling
C + I + O = Pleasurable relaxation
D + J + P = Crutch: tension reduction
E + K + Q = Craving: psychological addiction
F + L + R = Habit

Adapted from the National Cancer Institute. Why do you smoke? (No. 80-1822), DHEW, Bethesda, MD, 1980.

smoking are. Now think of what other behavior you could substitute. Experience your fear over the change. That feeling is the reason you have not given up smoking.

Change is scary. Changing from a smoker to a nonsmoker is scary. Get the suport you need. Organizations and friends were designed for this purpose. Remember that support is different for different people— get the amount and variety you need.

SELECTING YOUR CIGARETTE ALTERNATIVE

What your treatment options are depends upon what kind of smoker you are. The test in Table 4-5 was designed to provide you with a score on each of six factors that describe many people's smoking behavior. It is a means to help you identify what you use smoking for and what kind of satisfaction you think you get from smoking.

The first three factors—stimulation, handling, and pleasurable relaxation—all represent positive feelings people get from smoking. Substitutes involving a "wake-up" feeling and exciting activities need to be incorporated into your life. If you smoke for any of the reasons listed other than craving, you can give up smoking by tapering off gradually.

In substituting for stimulation, a brisk walk or exercise could be used whenever you have the urge to smoke. Handling a pen, doodling, or playing with some harmless object is better than handling cigarettes. Pleasurable social and physical activities can substitute for smoking to give you pleasurable relaxation. Many nurses use cigarette breaks to legitimize taking needed relaxation time.

Many smokers use the cigarette in moments of stress as a way to relieve discomfort. This reduction of stress is symptomatic relief. If you are this kind of smoker you may find it easy to stop when things are going well, but you may be tempted to start again at times of crisis.

You need to develop a plan to identify the skills necessary to cope effectively without cigarettes. Skills that help you deal with criticism and conflict are a vital part of the plan. Identifying and correcting behaviors that reduce your self-esteem are also very important.

"Craving," or psychological addiction, can only be dealt with by quitting "cold turkey." Support is essential to deal with the discomfort involved. Changing cigarettes to reduce the amount of nicotine inhaled will help with the physical withdrawal. Keeping yourself away from access to cigarettes until the craving is gone is often not practical, although this method is effective for many.

The habitual smoker no longer gets much satisfaction from a cigarette. Quitting in this case involves breaking habit patterns you have built up. Cutting down gradually may be effective if the conditions under which the cigarette is smoked are altered. The key to success here is *to become aware of each cigarette you smoke.* Ask yourself, "Do I really want this cigarette?"

THE PROCESS OF QUITTING

There is not one magic way for everybody to quit smoking; but there are a great many effective ways. If at first you don't succeed, quit and quit again!
Some good advice from a successful quitter.

This advice points out the essence of the successful resolution of tobacco dependence. A list of effective ways to quit smoking is compiled in a booklet entitled *Clearing the Air: A Guide to Quitting Smoking* (National Cancer Institute, 1981). The approaches include those most popular with ex-smokers.

Many smokers try to quit "cold turkey" without first reducing their smoking, designing a special program, or seeking professional help. However, most quitters find giving up cigarettes is easier when they replace smoking with new habits. *Clearing the Air* provides helpful hints and gimmicks other smokers have used to kick the habit. Suggestions are offered for each of the five stages of quitting:

1. Thinking about quitting:
2. Just before quitting
3. The day you quit
4. Immediately after quitting
5. Finding new habits.

In each of these stages important issues are addressed, such as cutting down, getting support, dealing with "the crazies," and gaining weight. Finally, other sources of information on quitting and professional programs are listed.

Since most of you reading this are in the "thinking about quitting" stage, some useful ideas in that stage are presented here. First, list all the reasons you want to quit. Think of reasons in addition to health reasons. Read this list every night before you go to bed. Second, when a negative thought about the difficulty of quitting arises, focus on a positive reason for quitting. A third idea is to condition yourself through moderate exercise, drinking more fluids, and getting appropriate rest. Then set a target date; perhaps you could celebrate your birthday or begin a vacation as a nonsmoker. Finally, involve someone else to support you in quitting.

The role of diet in reducing the desire to smoke was demonstrated in studies by Schachter (1981). This treatment method involves the concept of stress in relation to smoking. Schachter found that people who were heavy smokers had very acid urine, and highly acid urine promotes rapid nicotine removal from the body. These people smoked most when under the influence of alcohol and stress—two known urine acidizers. When they were given bicarbonate of soda to render their urine alkaline, the participants' desire to smoke was reduced significantly. Diet recommendations include selecting foods that are known to have an alkaline effect on the body and to avoid those foods that have an acid end reaction.

Vegetables and fruits are the best alkalizers. For example, dried lima beans, spinach, carrots, raisins, and figs all offer an alkaline effect of 11.0–42.0. Meats such as beef and chicken produce an acid effect of 11.0–14.0. You might begin giving up cigarettes by shifting your diet in an alkaline direction.

The best way to prevent tobacco dependence is to not start smoking. For obvious health reasons, you would do better to find other ways to increase your pleasure and stimulation and decrease your negative feelings. Strategies for lifestyle change in these areas are discussed throughout this book.

Dealing with Marijuana

Marijuana, known also as pot, grass, reefers, joints, Mary Jane, and hay, is actually the leaves and flowering spikes of a weed known as cannabis, or hemp. When dried it is smoked in the form of a cigarette that gives off a slightly pungent odor. The health risk is not as clear as the relationship between cigarette smoking and cancer. The clear risk involved in using marijuana is that you could be caught and have legal action brought against you. Depending on in which state you commit the crime, the punishment could range from a misdemeanor to years in jail. State laws are changing in the direction of decriminalization. In Alaska, there is no state law prohibiting the private possession and cultivation of marijuana for personal use. There continues to be much controversy over the legalization and use of marijuana (Zinberg, 1976).

The use of marijuana is widespread in the United States. Fifty-five million Americans—30 percent of the adult population—have tried marijuana, and 13 percent of the adult population uses it on a regular basis

(National Institute on Drug Abuse, 1979). Public opinion is moving in the direction of approving the regulation of marijuana for distribution. The regulation of marijuana should be founded on the same general principles governing alcohol and tobacco (National Academy of Sciences, 1982).

Even if marijuana use becomes legalized, you must consider other factors in deciding whether you want to use the drug. In one survey the main reason given for not using marijuana was lack of interest, not the possibility of prosecution (Drug Abuse Council, 1977). The effects you can expect from this drug depends upon the level of tetrahydrocannabinol in the marijuana and how frequently you use it. The more you use it and the heavier the dose, the more likely you are to develop physical and psychological problems. The results of studies comparing casual and heavy users showed a greater likelihood of multiple drug use, physical dependence on the drug, and poor work and social adjustment among heavy users. Casual use was defined as 1–4 times a month, and heavy use as 20–30 times a month (Mirin, Shapiro, Meyer, Pillard, & Fisher, 1971).

By now the acute effects of marijuana have been well elucidated. Subjective effects are an awareness of the subtlety of meaning in sight and sound and an increased vividness of sensual perception. An apparent slowing down of time is almost universally reported. Marijuana clearly impairs short-term memory, probably because it reduces the ability to concentrate.

A drug altering the body's natural functioning is likely to produce damaging effects if used repeatedly. Almost all reports of physical harm from cannabis use are based on observations of moderate to heavy, chronic use of the drug. Both Eastern and Western literature contain little evidence at this time that light to moderate use of cannabis has deleterious physical effects (U.S. Department of Health, Education, and Welfare, 1972).

TREATMENT

The treatment for marijuana users begins with abstinence. It takes about 7 days for the effects of one joint to clear. Since the drug is not physically addicting, a treatment plan to deal with withdrawal signs is not needed. In order to combat the psychological dependence, however, you must identify the need the drug has been fulfilling. The feeling of euphoria accompanying the high makes tension and stress disappear, and your increasing usage of marijuana can be as insidious as alcohol, tobacco, and other drug dependence.

In one study comparing casual and heavy users (Mirin et al., 1971), the casual users stressed the drug's pleasurable effects as their reason for smoking. The heavy users mentioned enhanced insight, the wish for union with some cosmic force, and the sense of harmony they felt when high as reasons for continued use. Perhaps this need for union could be better met by involvement with people and the development of the spiritual dimension. Real involvement with people can substitute for the pseudointimate atmosphere created by the use of drugs.

PREVENTION

Decriminalization of marijuana and the development of a reasonable drug policy would be a first step toward removing people from the illicit drug traffic milieu. Second, well-documented, nonbiased research needs to be conducted to determine the longterm effects of both casual and heavy marijuana use. If marijuana causes signficant damage, as alcohol invariably does, it may be discernible in the large number of people now in their late 30s and early 40s who have been using marijuana for 20 years.

The public needs to be alerted to alternative ways to cope with stress. Some of these ways are pleasurable escapes, while others involve direct problem-solving approaches.

Dealing with Stimulants

Stimulants are drugs, usually amphetamines, that increase alertness, reduce hunger, and provide a feeling of well-being. They are used to combat fatigue, curb appetite, and reduce a mild depression. The stimulants include cocaine, Benzedrine, Dexedrine, and "speed," or "crystal." Mild stimulants include caffeine and sugar-containing substances.

PHYSIOLOGICAL EFFECTS

According to current research findings, amphetamines increase the availability of noradrenalin at the nerve cell connections. They stimulate certain areas of the nervous system that control blood pressure, heart, and metabolic rates; the body is put in a general state of stress, as if it were extremely threatened. Amphetamines artificially intensify and prolong such stimulation, keeping the body in a state of tension for prolonged periods of time.

In the United States, approximately one-fourth of all medical prescriptions for mood-altering drugs are for stimulants, mainly amphetamines (National Clearing House for Drug Abuse, 1981). Limiting these drugs to availability only by prescription did not end their misuse. Today their abuse is a major medical and social problem.

Amphetamines are used for two reasons related to stress—depression and appetite control. Some individuals suffering from burnout use this drug to gain the sense of power, self-confidence, and exhilaration artificially created by amphetamines. Even more people use this drug to help them combat the problem of being overweight. Having eaten to calm their anxiety, they then turn to "uppers" to suppress their appetite and deal with their feelings of inferiority associated with their excess pounds.

The consequences of using stimulants in the short term are hyperalertness, increased short-term performance, and a rapidly increasing tolerance. Occasional users take the drug to exert themselves beyond their physiological limits. The individuals who are drug dependent take amounts far beyond the average dose of 15–30 mg. Their dose is 75–100 mg daily, and the short-term effects are a high level of excitation. The name "speed freak" is associated with this state of high activity.

Long-term use of high doses of speed can result in liver and brain damage. Many users suffer from malnutrition and vitamin deficiencies. Some develop anorexia nervosa from using amphetamines for dieting. Their resulting impulsive, unpredictable behavior tends to lead to a deterioration in their social relationships. Their judgment, personality, and health deteriorate with long-term use. The physiological addiction and psychological dependence on stimulants, in many cases, needs medical and psychiatric treatment for effective and safe withdrawal. Treatment begins when you stop the drug. If you suspect a colleague is abusing stimulants, you may want to watch for some of the behaviors listed in Table 4-4.

TREATMENT: GETTING HIGH NATURALLY

You are most likely to use this drug to deal with life problems if you are frequently apathetic and depressed, unable to feel or enjoy the natural "turn-ons" or "highs" that others find in normal experience, and, perhaps, unable to relate easily to others.

Treatment would therefore be focused on facilitating the development of satisfying interpersonal relationships. Getting high on people and your own activities will allow you to experience the joy of relating and the self-confidence derived from achievement. A considerable amount of social and psychological support may be required to break this addiction because the fatigue and depression you experience when you stop the drug are so severe that you may be strongly tempted to return to the drug. If you are using amphetamines to lose weight, I suggest you see the section on dealing with food (p. 93) for alternative ways of losing weight.

Cocaine is another powerful stimulant that helps the mind forget. It is also in fashion, replacing the more commonplace pot. In snorting cocaine, the person experiences the ecstatic high of amphetamines in one shot. The long-term effects of heavy use are bleeding from the nose and hyperactivity; some psychotic symptoms have been reported. Treatment involves creating experiences that foster natural highs and genuine involvement with people.

Dealing with Mild Stimulants: Caffeine and Sugar

Two mild stimulants, caffeine and sugar, are often overlooked in analyzing people's use of drugs to cope with depression. There may even be group pressure to conform by having coffee and a sugar donut on work breaks; however, work breaks were designed as a time to relax. Caffeine and sugar do not create a relaxation response—they are drugs (defined as substances that have an effect on the mind and body) disguised as food. They are mind-altering chemicals.

"Refined sugar overstimulates the production of insulin and alkaline digestive juices, interferes with the absorption of proteins, calcium, and many other minerals, and retards the growth of valuable intestinal bacteria" (Davis, 1965, p. 311). This overstimulation of the body also affects the mind, causing temporary alertness. The functioning of the brain and nervous tissue is more sensitively dependent on the rate of chemical reactions than the functioning of any other organ. Therefore, the stimulation induced by sugar can have a profound effect on mental clarity.

Caffeine stimulation—an accepted "morning fix" for many people— has come under increasing attack as studies on coronary disease proliferate. One study showed that even a single cup of coffee, acting as a stress, causes a prompt rise in blood fats and cholesterol (Keys, 1957). Coffee, alcohol, and strong tea increase the amount and concentration of stomach acid. Caffeine-containing drinks such as coffee, tea, and cola, as well as chocolate containing caffeine, all trigger the body into a stress response.

Our dietary habits play a major role in preventing and treating stress. More often than most people realize, they use food as a way to dampen their tension and anxiety. Food, much like alcohol or other tranquilizing drugs, can be abused as a tension reducer. Overconsumption of the chief tranquilizing food—sugar products—has made obesity a major health problem in the United States. The average man is 14 pounds overweight and the average female is 21 pounds overweight. Obesity is increasing in frequency, and so is diabetes. The number of diagnosed diabetics is 6 million, and an estimated 4 million are undiagnosed. The disease is increasing annually at the rate of 6 percent a year. The pancreas becomes overburdened by the average American's consumption of 128 pounds of sugar a year (Lecos, 1980); therefore, it quits effectively converting the sucrose to glucose. Moreover, the stress-triggering mechanisms induced by sugar consumption affect the pancreas. It is little wonder that diabetes and hypoglycemia are so prevalent in the United States.

GIVING UP YOUR A.M. AND P.M. FIX

Abstinence is the first step in the treatment of sugar and caffeine abuse. The most dramatic stories about changing diet usually concern sugar. The following is a story told by a head nurse in a stress management seminar:

First of all, this experience is going to be shared here only because if anyone of you are willing to go the distance and get off sugar, I want you to know that at least one person in the world understands what you're going through. For those who don't experience withdrawal from sugar as bad as I am about to describe, just thank God that you are one of the chosen few to have an easier experience. Simply put, I swore I had caught the flu—aching joints, temperature 100, general malaise, nauseated in general for 3 days. I thought this was the worst flu I had ever experienced. I called up the doctor who was a nutritional expert and had counseled me about the problems of my sugar intake and the cleansing process. I told him I had caught the flu and named the symptoms. He said, "I want you to know that you are experiencing withdrawal signs." "Withdrawal signs, why didn't you tell me I would have these symptoms?" I screamed. "Would you have done it?" he replied. "Yes, and I wouldn't have had to think I had the flu." He still doesn't tell people, and I tell people and they can't believe me, so I guess it doesn't matter.

I wish you the courage to know you are doing something very important for your body and for your emotional state. I no longer have the emotional ups and downs. I can now control my eating. I have stopped binging. And anything that makes you feel like you have the flu when it leaves your body can't be good for your body. A few more words about withdrawal—you may get psychological and craving signs rather than physical signs. Hang in there, it diminishes by the fourth day.

This story may sound dramatic, but there are many stories like this. Some other people experience the transition much more slowly and quietly.

Going "off" sugar does not mean substituting an equal amount of honey, maple syrup, or saccharine. If you do that, you have done the equivalent of what heroin addicts do when they switch to methadone. Saccharine is a substitute for refined sugar like methadone is for heroin. All are drugs. Maple sugar and honey in amounts equivalent to sugar still overstimulate your pancreas. A minimal use of honey can satisfy your sweet tooth and allow stable blood sugar levels.

Substituting for caffeine products involves several alternatives. Natural fruit juices are substitutes for colas; decaffeinated coffee, Cafix (coffee-like grain drink), or herb teas can substitute for coffee and tea; and carob is a substitute for chocolate. All these substitutions can be added gradually to your diet as you switch from caffeine products to natural foods.

Some sleepiness, fatigue, and possibly headaches may accompany withdrawal from caffeine. If you are consuming four cups or more a day, you may experience some shakiness with sudden withdrawal. With gradual elimination the withdrawal signs are less intense.

PREVENTING THE NEED FOR ARTIFICIAL
STIMULATION

In order to avoid the use of artificial stimulants you will need to lead
a life balanced with risk-taking excitement and stability. All humans have
a need for some level of stimulation to their central nervous system; the
degree of intensity and the amount vary with the individual's make-up. If
your life is not exciting enough, then you need to decide and plan for
some adventure. White-water rafting, opening night at the theater, giving
a surprise party, or simply trying something new all contribute to the
natural excitement of life.

If you are using stimulants to exert yourself beyond your physiological limits, consider whether it is worth the price you are paying. Overworking is both a cause and a consequence of burnout. Your body, running at full throttle over a period of time, will show signs of wear and
tear. Our stress response was designed for handling emergencies; to place
your body in a state of continuous emergency is bound to play havoc with
your health.

Dealing with Food

Experts now recognize the "binge syndrome" as an eating disorder
affecting many millions of people. Most people can identify with overeating occassionally; however, many people are not aware of the emotional
connection. We must have food for nourishment, but for most people
food means a lot more than the necessary diet.

Food has different meanings for different people. One person's internal response to eating a sugar donut might be "Sweets for the sweet. You
were such a good little girl." Another person's, however, might be
"Don't eat the donut it is full of sugar. You know how you feel on
sugar." One colleague of mine calls the former type "El Fatso" messages.
These "El Fatso" messages encourage eating and in many cases result in
binge eating. It is important that you become aware of these messages in
order to understand why you eat what you eat. For example, some foods
create a feeling of well-being because the hot food is associated with
warmth and security. Hot oatmeal or hot cider conjure up images, messages, and feelings about food.

Foods are used as emotional tools with children. All too often, dessert is given as a reward for good behavior or for cleaning off your plate.
Withholding of food as a form of punishment can lead to rebellious night
eating. With almost everyone subjected to years of parental and advertising messages about food, it is no wonder that emotional eating is so
prevalent. Habituation to processed and refined foods full of sugar and

chemicals also contributes to many people using food for more than suste-
nance. Finally, modern-day stress that taxes an already unhealthy body
can lead to emotional compulsive eating. Some people use food to numb
themselves to their emotional pain and then forget that the pain has
anything to do with the eating of the food. Although this sounds like an
addiction process, food is not a true physiological trigger. The drive to eat
certain foods is an obsessive-compulsive emotional response. Your craving for chocolate cake may feel like an addict's craving for heroin, but
your need exists basically on an emotional level.

The problem with overeating as a method of coping is that it leaves
tell-tale evidence. This method of coping with pain, grief, excess energy,
or negative thoughts could be costing you heavily in deteriorating health.
The emotional eater swallows feelings, pushing them down with food.

DIAGNOSING OVEREATING

The quiz in Table 4-6 will help you find out what causes you to
overeat and how much of an emotional overeater you are. This increased
self-knowledge is meant to help you solve your overeating problem.

CHANGING EATING PATTERNS

If your score is high enough to indicate problems, read *Fat Is a
Feminist Issue* by Orbach (1978) and *Winning the Diet Wars* by Merzen
(1980), and attend Overeaters Anonymous meetings.* All three of these
sources will support you in understanding your overeating and can help
you learn to eat like a normal person. A nurse in a workshop once said,
"It took 34 years for me to admit I was addicted to food; cigarettes and
alcohol were a breeze compared to admitting my food addiction."

Treatment for overeating is even more complicated than treatment
for alcoholism or drug addiction. With alcohol and most drugs treatment
is a matter of complete withdrawal, it is not the daily issue of moderation,
as it is with food. Food, especially if it contains sugar, is an over-the-
counter tranquilizer.

Guilt over the intake of food is a constant issue for the emotional
over-eater. Life becomes filled with thinking about what you eat and
what you do not eat. You are either resisting or giving into the temptation of food. Seems similar to alcoholism or drug addiction, doesn't it?
All three substances are abused to reduce the stress of life.

In order to deal with emotional over-eating you first need to understand your binging pattern. Keep a journal of when, where, and why you

---

*For information or a local group contact, write or call Overeaters Anonymous World
Service Office, 2190 190th Street, Torrance, CA 90504, (213) 320-7941.

overeat. By recognizing your vulnerable times you can take either preventive or preparative action. Second, focus on directing your thoughts. Instead of focusing negatively—e.g., "I won't binge"—focus on saying and imagining only positive things. Picturing yourself eating normal amounts and telling yourself that you eat normally are two ways to direct your thoughts.

The third approach is behaviorally oriented to help free you of negatively reinforcing behavior and replace it with positive eating habits. Exercising in moderation helps relieve the tension likely to send you off on a binge. Saving 200 calories a day, beginning Monday, allows you 1,000 calories for that party Saturday night. This behavioral approach to handling social eating situations reduces the strain of being in a situation with a lot of food. In fact, there is another way to control your portions— never eat out of a bag; remove the portion you intend to eat and put the rest away.

Some other useful ideas deal with changing behaviors related to weighing and binging patterns. Stay off the scale! Weigh yourself a maximum of once every 2 weeks. Most people weigh themselves entirely too often; if they have not lost weight they become guilty, which triggers overeating. To motivate yourself further, add up the cost of all the foods you have cut out of one week. Keep this binge money in a special fund to buy yourself a gift. Learn to eat "just one" through focusing on the taste and sensation of the food. Anything more is just repetition.

The fourth part of treatment involves asking for help from friends, a counselor, and organizations. Reaching out for support instead of food is difficult for most overeaters. Asking for help is essential to being able to control emotional eating.

Organizations such as Overeaters Anonymous have been helping overeaters loose weight and change their eating patterns. Overeaters Anonymous has helped compulsive overeaters through a comprehensive program that focuses on three levels: physical, emotional, and spiritual. The principles of daily living, or the "12 steps," form the spiritual basis of the program and are identical to those used in Alcoholics Anonymous.

Six tools are also given to aid the practice of the steps. Abstinence from compulsive overeating is supported by a food plan being chosen and adhered to. Many overeaters have to abstain completely from refined carbohydrates due to the cravings they stimulate. Meetings, telephone calls, and sponsorship all contribute the support necessary to deal with the problem. The fifth tool is literature to reinforce the program, and the final tool is anonymity, allowing for free expression. All the tools are important in dealing with emotional overeating.

Overeaters Anonymous speaks to the issue of the feelings involved in obsessive-compulsive eating and Weight Watchers provides a reasonable

Table 4-6
ARE YOU AN EMOTIONAL OVEREATER?

1. Do you feel compelled to eat something after you have had an argument with someone who means a lot to you?
2. Do you need to eat when you feel worried, depressed, or tense?
3. Is your idea of a "reward" a special food, going out to eat, or splurging on a calorie-rich dessert or starchy ethnic food?
4. You are on a diet. Your hostess or a friend you are lunching with insists that you eat some forbidden, high-calorie food like a sundae or a slice of pie. How often do you give in to this kind of pressure—perhaps even with a secret feeling of relief, because you now have an excuse to break or bend your diet?
5. You have sampled a high-calorie food or a food forbidden on your diet. Does that "sample taste" set you off on a major or minor binge?
6. When you walk by a bakery or a candy shop do you give in to the temptation to go in and buy sweets?
7. Do you eat foods that you know are "bad" for you?
8. Did your parents reward you with sweets?
9. How frequently do you feel that if you eat something, you will feel better?
10. Do you gulp down your food instead of chewing slowly and savoring its taste?
11. Do you ever feel surprised that you have eaten so much without really noticing what went into your mouth—just shoveled it in without thinking?
12. How often do you put yourself on a diet to lose weight and then find yourself breaking the diet rather quickly and uncontrollably?
13. Do you have eating binges that last for several days at a time?
14. Do you plan ahead of time to have secret/solo eating binges?
15. Do you find yourself eating even though you are not really hungry?
16. Do you hide foods, so that you can keep them for yourself alone?
17. You feel really full. Do you eat anyway?
18. Do you eat standing up?
19. Do you find that there are some foods that you just cannot stop eating?
20. Do you feel guilty about your eating habits and eating patterns?
21. Some people eat to live; others live to eat. How often do you find yourself "living for the sake of eating"?
22. Do you feel you are struggling to keep your appetite under control?
23. You cannot concentrate on an important assignment. You have a snack, because you will think better after you have eaten. How often have you done this?
24. Are there periods of time when eating is one of the major joys in your life?
25. How often do you think about your weight or your eating patterns of diet, binge, diet, binge?

26. Do you scan the latest fad and wonder diets, looking for some kind of miracle solution to your weight and eating problems?
27. Are you ashamed of the way your body looks?
28. Have you avoided seeing old friends because you were ashamed of how much weight you have put on?
29. Have you ever postponed buying new clothes because you are ashamed of your shape/size/weight and hate the way clothes look on you?
30. Do your overeating habits make you feel that you are lacking in self-control and hence are an inferior person?
31. Are you kinder or nicer to other people than you are to yourself?

How to score
Assign one number to each question, according to the following scale:

1 = Never
2 = Seldom
3 = Occasionally
4 = Frequently
5 = Always

Add up the numbers for a total score, and see below for the interpretation of your score.

51 points or less. You are not at all compulsive about your eating habits. You see food as a requirement for your body. Your eating habits probably have little relationship to your moods.

52–74 points. Emotions play a small role in your eating. When it comes to choosing what, when, and how much to eat you are only mildly affected by your emotions.

75–87 points. The emotional and compulsive components of your eating behavior are in the average range. When you are calm, eating is a sensual pleasure; under pressure you may undereat or overeat. Your emotions affect how much you eat.

88–119 points. The emotional and compulsive components of your eating behavior are greater than average. You want to eat when triggered by a strong emotion. You go on and off diets, and controlling your weight is a struggle. Your idea of an enjoyable time is a good meal in pleasant company.

Over 199 points. You are a compulsive overeater. You eat for emotional reasons you may not be aware of. You are using food as an anesthetic to cope with life's problems. You spend a considerable amount of time thinking about food. You are either on a diet, feeling you should be, or feeling guilty for having lapsed off one.

If you have scored over 88, it is very important to be kinder to yourself. What you have considered your lack of willpower is actually the result of your emotions and compulsions regarding food.

Adapted from Merzen, M. *Winning the Diet Wars*. New York: Harcourt Brace Jovanovich, 1980.

diet to follow.* Most of you know what to eat; the answer is beyond nutritional information. I do not want to underemphasize the importance of an effective nutritional regime like that of Weight Watchers, however, most of you will need more help than a once-a-week Weight Watchers meeting will offer.

ANTIADDICTION APPROACHES: NATURAL NUTRITION AND A SUPPORTIVE ENVIRONMENT

Preventing addictions involves finding natural ways to keep anxiety at a profitable level, not allowing everyday stress to tip the balance into anxiety or depression. The goal is to keep the internal world of the body and the mind comfortable and to create an external environment supportive of good health.

Natural highs and a sense of inner calmness are equivalent. In order to achieve this state, the body and mind need to be relaxed and focused. Once your body and mind are balanced you will feel no need for drugs to reduce stress, basically because you will not experience the extreme emotional and physical fluctuations that drugs are designed to curb.

One of four natural methods to accomplish this balance was mentioned in Chapter 2—physical fitness. Exercising creates a calming effect on the body that lasts far beyond the 15–30 minutes of exercise. The mind, having focused on an activity, also is calmer. Studies suggest that this effect is probably due to the release of endorphins, natural morphine-like substances produced by the body (Strahinich, 1982).

Meditation, another natural method mentioned in Chapter 2, is key in reducing the stress and the need for drugs. Some studies of meditation used to treat hypertension showed a 19mm Hg reduction in the systolic and 4.4 mm Hg difference in the diastolic blood pressure (Benson, 1973; Benson et al., 1974). In a study of 1,450 drug users, marijuana use decreased from 78 percent of the sample to 37 percent after 6 months of meditation, and to 12 percent at 12 months (Benson & Wallace, 1972). In another study, after 22 months of meditation, the drinkers in the sample decreased from 60 percent to 25 percent; the number of cigarette smokers decreased from 48 percent to 16 percent (Benson, 1974).

Physiological changes occur with meditation: decreased oxygen consumption, lower heart rate, and lower muscle tension have been registered. You feel calmer; a calm you have created yourself, rather than a drug-induced calm, increases your sense of self-esteem and self-control.

---

*For information or a local group contact, write or call Weight Watchers International, 800 Community Drive, Manhasset, NY 11031, (516) 627-9200.

The two natural methods of achieving inner calm elaborated upon in this chapter are changing your diet and altering your environment. First the effect of your nutritional state on your level of stress and tension is examined. "We are what we eat," is true in many ways. Preventing body and mind stress involves examining and altering some of your dietary practices. At the end of the chapter is a short section on designing your environment for stress reduction.

Natural Nutrition

Begin by testing yourself on your knowledge of nutrition—you may surprise yourself. This is not a nursing school test on nutrition; you know those answers. These are questions about lifestyle nutrition and the effects of eating what you do. Read each of the nine statements below and consider whether it is true or false. Then read the answer and the brief discussion of each topic. This is important nutritional information that you should take into consideration in changing your eating habits.

1. One and one-half cups of beans (or peas) or 4 cups of rice has the same amount of usable protein as a 6–7 ounce steak.

This statement is true. Even more interesting is the fact that by combining the beans and rice you increase the usable protein to that in a 13–19 ounce steak. Grains plus beans can provide over 40 percent more usable protein than if you ate them separately (Lappe, 1975).

2. Tea has a significant amount of caffeine, like coffee and cola.

This statement is true. Most people are unaware of the significant effects of caffeine on the body and mind (Ferguson, 1982). Take a look at how much caffeine exists in the products listed in Table 4-7, and you may think twice about that second cup.

3. There is little difference in the vitamin C and the vitamin A content of fresh, frozen, and canned fruits and vegetables.

This statement is false. For example, on the average, fresh orange juice contains 130 mg vitamin C per 8-ounce glass. Frozen juice varies depending on the type of oranges, method of extraction, and length of time it has been stored. Little ascorbic acid is destroyed when foods are quickly frozen, but losses of up to 90 percent may occur within 1 hour after the food has thawed. Much vitamin C is lost in the soaking and boiling process of canning.

4. The average American eats 128 pounds of sugar per year.

This statement is true. According to the U.S. Department of Agriculture (USDA), the sugar consumption in the United States has been relatively stable for more than 50 years: it is now approximately 100 pounds a year per person. However, these figures do not reflect the growing impact of a variety of corn sweeteners now in use. When all these are taken into account, USDA figures show a rise in per capita consumption from 122 pounds in 1970 to 128 pounds in 1978 (Lecos, 1980).

5.   White flour is really no different than wheat flour.

This statement is false. Wheat, rye, and buckwheat all still have the wheat germ hull. This kernal is the most nutritious part, full of minerals and vitamins. In white flour, the kernal (vitamins and minerals) has been destroyed by bleaching. To make "enriched" white flour, 4 vitamins and minerals (of the original 20 before bleaching) are put back in. (Only good advertising could sell us on "enriched" white bread!)

6.   Hot dogs and luncheon meats, despite their nitrates, do not contribute to cancer.

This statement is false. If the only time you eat a hot dog is when the Phillies win the pennant, you need not worry. However, if you eat luncheon meat sandwiches for lunch and salami for snacks, you could be asking for trouble. Nitrates and nitrites can combine with other chemicals in your body to form nitrosamines, which, in small amounts, can contribute to cancer.

7.   The average vegetarian diet provides a sufficient amount of fiber.

This statement is true. It is not true of the average American diet, which contains 6 g fiber daily, whereas 20 g is recommended. Two tablespoons of bran provides 6 g fiber. Four slices of wheat bread provides 1.6 g, and 4 ounces of beans provides 5 g. Add an apple, a pear, and a cup of peas and you have 20 g a day. Perhaps now you can see why most people do not get their recommended roughage for a day. Bran is the greatest natural nutritional cure for constipation ("Fiber," 1980).

8.   Your pancreas actually responds differently to the sugar in an apple compared to that in a sugar donut.

This statement is true. Sugar Blues (1975) talks about the metabolic disruption that occurs with refined sugar. When we take refined sugar it largely escapes chemical processing in our bodies. The sucrose passes directly to the intestines where it is absorbed into the blood, raising the glucose level and destroying the precise balance of glucose and oxygen. Fruit, on the other hand, buffers the absorption of its own natural sugars (frutose) because of its high fiber content. Fruit provides the kind of gradual and usable energy boost that a candy bar cannot. Do not panic your pancreas with a 300-calorie candy bar; instead, eat three medium-sized apples, or $1\frac{1}{2}$ quarts of strawberries. After all, they have the same number of calories!

9. The average American consumes $2-2\frac{1}{2}$ teaspoons of salt a day ($8\frac{1}{2}$ pounds a year).

This statement is true. The USDA reports that the average person consumes 4–5 g ($2\frac{1}{2}$ teaspoons) salt a day. The National Research Council estimated in 1980 that an adequate and safe sodium intake is 1.1–1.3 g a day (Fenner, 1980). Do not ignore the hidden sodium in processed foods when you are trying to reduce your salt intake. Check the labels!

The nutrition literature repeatedly makes seven major recommendations to improve the health of your body and mind:

1. Eliminate all refined sugars and refined flour from your diet. Due to various refining procedures, as much as 40 percent of the food value in the 3,500 calories the average American eats each day is lost.
2. Increase the fiber content of your diet to at least 20 g a day.
3. Reduce the amount of fat in your diet to a maximum of 30 percent of your total calorie intake. Use no more than three teaspoons of unrefined vegetable oils a day and reduce the intake of high-fat products, such as meat and cheese.
4. Increase the amount of fresh vegetables you eat to three or four servings a day. One vegetable should be raw, or eat a vegetable salad. Other vegetable servings should include dark-green or yellow varieties.
5. Eliminate coffee, tea, cola, and chocolate. All these substances contain caffeine. Caffeine is a central nervous system stimulant that quickens your metabolism by about 10 percent. Your muscles react by tensing up, your stomach and urinary tract overproduce, and your heart and lung blood vessels dilate. Thiamine (vitamin B_1), essential to the health of your nervous system, is destroyed. Your body builds a tolerance to caffeine rather quickly—the more you drink the more you need. If you need a stimulant (without a built-in tolerance), try increasing your body's output of adrenalin by running in place. Splashing your face with cold water will also wake you up.
6. Increase the amount of complex carbohydrates you eat. Fresh pineapple, strawberries, cantaloupe, and blueberries are great desserts; you can even add walnuts and oats. Whole grains—brown rice, bulgar wheat, whole-grain cereals, and nuts—not only add bulk and B vitamins, but also produce satiety.

Table 4-7
CAFFEINE IS THE CULPRIT (AND IT'S NOT ONLY IN COFFEE)

Source	Approximate Caffeine	
Beverages		
Brewed coffee	100–150	mg/cup
Instant coffee	86–99	mg/cup
Tea	60–75	mg/cup
Decaffeinated coffee	2–4	mg/cup
Cola drinks	40–60	mg/glass
Over-the-counter analgesics		
Anacin, aspirin compound, Bromo-Seltzer	32	mg/tablet
Cope, Easy-Mens, Empirin Compound, Midol	32	mg/tablet
Vanquish	32	mg/tablet
Excedrin	60	mg/tablet
Pre-Mens	66	mg/tablet
Many over-the-counter cold preparations	30	mg/tablet
Many over-the-counter stimulants	100	mg/tablet

Reprinted from Shimer, P. Pros and cons of coffee: Caffeine is the culprit—And its not just in coffee. *Executive Fitness Newsletter,* 1979, *10*(17), 4. With permission.

7. Get more of your protein from plant sources and fish and less from meat. Here are some facts to support your stopping or decreasing your meat intake: It takes 16 pounds of grain for a steer to produce 1 pound of meat; 90 percent of all our barley, corn, and oats are consumed by our livestock; meat has repeatedly been found to contain toxins due to livestock practices; and meat has a high fat content, which often creates digestive complications (Lappe, 1975).

Although we are historically omnivorous (both plant and meat eating), our anatomical equipment—teeth, jaws, digestive system—favors a plant diet. The American Dietetic Association notes that "most of mankind for much of history has subsisted on near-vegetarian diets" (Lappe, 1975). In the United States the focus on meat is less than 100 years old. It is probably a result of the affluence of the 20th century. The average American eats more than 200 pounds of meat, poultry, and seafood annually; in 1940 the figure was 150 pounds (Lappe, 1975).

Most animal proteins are complete. Two or more incomplete proteins can be combined to form a complete protein. Many combinations are given in *Recipes for a Small Planet* (Ewald, 1973). Once you learn the basic combinations, planning meals is easy.

The basis for these recommendations is the *Dietary Goals for the United States* (U.S. Senate Select Committee, 1977). In Table 4-8, the average American diet is compared with the recommended diet. As you begin to change your diet, keep these percentages in mind. A book that would be helpful is *Diet and Disease* by Martin and Tenenbaum (1980). You will probably be surprised when you notice how much of your diet comes from fat and refined carbohydrate.

Why is it so difficult to get adequate nutrition today? Refined and processed foods are part of the answer. Since sugar provides about 20 percent of your calories, you must get 80 percent by selecting foods that supply the other nutrients. If you are also trying to lose weight, the chances are not good that you will get adequate vitamins and minerals. Until the trend toward refined and processed foods is reversed, supplements will probably be necessary.

Another reason is that the cultivating, harvesting, shipping, processing, and cooking of foods today create foods with poor vitamin quality. Unless you have your own organic garden and do your own canning and freezing you are likely to need supplements. Vitamin and mineral supplements are not substitutes for good nutrition habits; they are additions to a diet favoring natural foods.

Use of Vitamin Supplements

The question of whether or not to take vitamins always arises when nutrition is being discussed. Some experts say "no," other say "yes." Even those who recommend them disagree about when and how much to take.

According to Linus Pauling, vitamin C helps prevent many diseases, and according to other sources vitamin C is grossly overrated. Most views lie somewhere between the two extremes. Vitamin C is most often recommended for all smokers, heavy meat eaters, people living in high-pollution areas, and people with respiratory problems.

How much should you take? The only reliable way to answer that question involves testing. You would be given doses of oral Vitamin C over a period of time and your urine would be tested to see when you began

Table 4-8
COMPARISON OF AVERAGE AMERICAN DIET AND
RECOMMENDED DIET

Nutrient	Average Intake (%)	Recommended Intake (%)
Fat	42	30
Saturated	16	10
Monounsaturated	19	10
Polyunsaturated	7	10
Protein	12	12
Carbohydrates	46	58
Complex	22 ⎫	48
Natural	6 ⎭	
Refined	18	10

Adapted from *Dietary Goals for the United States* (U.S. Senate Select Committee, 1977).

excreting Vitamin C. The dose just under that at which you began to excrete the Vitamin C would be the correct one for you. This is expensive and it is not easy to find someone to do this testing. The amounts mentioned below are the average of the amounts recommended by three holistic health centers in New York, Pennsylvania, and California.

For vitamin C, 1000 mg a day was the average recommended amount. Vitamin C and vitamin B are often combined (one currently available product is Stress Tabs). These vitamins are the ones most depleted during the body's stress reaction. Vitamin B, like vitamin C, is necessary to help the body cope. The vitamin B group is necessary for enzyme reactions and for the nervous system. Vitamin B helps in nerve conduction and digestion. It is found normally in whole-grain breads, eggs, liver, cereals, and some fresh vegetables. Since most Americans do not eat much of these foods, subclinical cases of deficiency are frequently found. (See Davis, 1954 p. 65, for the tongue test for deficiency). The quantity of vitamin B supplement needs to be increased gradually, otherwise the sudden shock to your intestinal system will give you flatulence. The average daily amount recommended was 50 mg.

Basically, the B vitamins—thiamine, niacin, riboflavin, vitamin B_{12}, etc.—are a complex, which means they work together and they generally occur together in the same foods. However, each B vitamin has some specific functions and a deficiency causes problems. For example, if you are on the birth control pill Pyrodoxine, 500 mg vitamin B_6 a day is recommended. Low levels of B_6 have been repeatedly found in the blood tests of women on oral contraceptives. If you are a vegetarian, you may need to take a vitamin B_{12} supplement, unless you use brewer's yeast. Vitamin B_{12} is found almost exclusively in foods of animal origin. Antacids destroy vitamin B in the stomach, as do antibiotics in the digestive tract. Many other drugs destroy vitamins. *Vitamins*, by Adams (1978), provides information on all vitamins.

The recommendations for other vitamins and minerals vary from none to hundreds of times the Recommended Daily Allowance. Because vitamin C and vitamin B are water soluable, there is no risk of overdosing. Many of you probably have some deficiencies in vitamins and minerals. Updating your knowledge on the importance of adequate nutrition and supplements could help you choose a healthier lifestyle. Remember that vitamin supplements are not meant to replace a healthy diet.

Designing Your Environment for Stress Reduction

Environment, according to *Webster's* is "circumstances, objects, or conditions by which you are surrounded." The world around you is your environment—your universe, your planet, your city, your neighborhood, your house, and your place of work. From the largest dimensions of your world to its smallest parameter is your environment. Your environment has an impact on you and you have an impact on your environment.

Close your eyes and visualize the environment of your planet. What do you like and what do you not like? Opportunities for being a part of the natural environment may enhance your life. Think of your neighborhood, house, and place of work. What do you find pleasant? What is unpleasant?

To design a less stressful environment, you need to consider your sensory dimensions—sight, sound, smell, hearing, and touch. Begin with your home environment. Walk in your front door and take a slow tour through your house or apartment. Look at the arrangement of the rooms, the colors, the lighting. Consider the type of environment you want to create around you—relaxed, quiet, sunny. The use of colors and lighting can create entirely different effects. You may want to invest in a course in interior decorating given by a major local department store or high school. Through such courses you can learn the basics of creating the type of home environment you want.

Claus and Bailey (1980) note the effect of colors on patients and nurses. Here are a few suggestions for making your work environment more pleasing: a philodendron plant (very hard to kill, even with no light; however, they are poisonous to children); colorful contrast paper; pictures posters you have framed; scraps of wallpaper (to wallpaper stores scraps are actually unusable rolls). Develop a new system for organizing charts, medicines, dressings—you name it, and it can be reorganized to be less stressful. List some ideas for your work unit.

You can influence your broader environment too in ways that reduce stress in the neighborhood or on the planet. Pollution, nuclear hazards, and crime are not only your neighbors' problems. In our world system we are all affected directly or indirectly by rising taxes and pollution.

When suggestions are made for changing the earth's environment, people usually say "What I would do can't make a difference," or "When big industry starts, I'll start." With these defeatist or self-righteous attitudes, it is no wonder our environment is such a mess. Put your excuse aside for a minute, and with as much openness as you can, pick one of the following measures to make a positive contribution to your environment:

Recycle papers
Recycle glass
Join a food co-op
Be a Big Brother or Big Sister
Create a "clean up your neighborhood day"
Contribute to your local paper on health issues.

Add your own ideas to this list. Contribute some time, effort, money to making your neighborhood and planet a healthier and prettier place to live.

Your outdoors, home, and work environments affect your level of tension. Making your environment as tranquil or as exciting as you need it to be will help you to reach these states without abusing drugs or food. Remember that the design of your environment profoundly affects your physical and emotional state. Taking care of yourself includes being more involved in the design of your environment.

You have now identified how you use drugs and food to cope with stress. Too often addictions are not thought of as stress-coping mechanisms and are allowed to go unchecked. Having identified your particular coping strategy, you can begin to take treatment and preventive steps.

In Chapters 2–4, the focus has been on physical, psychological, and behavioral causes, consequences, and strategies for coping with stress. In the next chapter the focus shifts to your work environment as a direct source of stress.

5

Work Strategies: Clarifying and Changing Sources of Work Stress

STRESS AS A RESULT OF THE ROLE OF THE NURSE

Finding solutions for work stressors is the dual responsibility of the organization and the individual nurse. Our national organization of nurses—the ANA—is also actively involved on the political front to change nursing into a less stressful profession. Nurses working on task forces and commissions are making our needs known.

In this chapter the focus is on what you, as a nurse, can do about work stress. First, the reasons the role itself is stressful are explored. Next, self-assessments are provided for you to diagnose the internal and external factors that contribute to your stress. The bulk of the chapter is concerned with what you can do for yourself to treat and prevent burnout.

High levels of stress are caused by the nursing role itself; the nursing shortage is one result of this. Some reasons for this stress are clear.

Older Patient Population

The role of nurses will change as the population changes and as the health care system changes. By the year 2000 it is predicted that our population will increase to 260 million (an increase of 40 million people), and this will include a large increase in the number of people over 65 years old. The continuing increase in the number of aged persons will have a major impact on hospitals, since the per capita cost of health care for persons over 65 is three times that of the rest of the population (McCarty, 1982).

Since 1969, when the nursing care differential was adopted, studies have shown that the average inpatient over 65 years of age requires more intensive nursing care than the average under-65 inpatient. Four studies (cited by the American Hospital Association, 1981) have shown cost differentials for Medicare patients ranging from 9 to 15 percent. One study, conducted in the 1,128-bed Greenville Hospital System (Greenville, S.C.) in 1979, found that, on the average, aged patients required 7.63 average hours of routine nursing care per day, while younger patients needed 6.86 hours per day. This is 1 extra hour of care a day. In 1982, 11.5 percent of the population was over 65, but by 2000 17–18 percent of the population will be that old. Other statistics on the elderly show that one of nine Americans is over 65, and in 50 years this ratio could be one of five. Furthermore, 25 percent of all elderly persons are admitted to hospitals (as inpatients or outpatients) at least once a year, and the average hospital patient today is more ill, and slightly older than the average patient in 1972 ("Decreased Federal Spending," 1981; "Eight and One-Half Percent Differential," 1981). The patient population hospital nurses will be caring for is likely to continue to be more ill as hospitals pressured with cost factors and limited bed space will be able to serve only the most ill.

Changes in Job Setting

Nurses' roles are changing and new roles for nurses have opened. In 1974, 80 percent of the nurses worked in hospitals; today 62 percent work in hospitals. The grim data on the current nurse shortage indicate that of the 1.4 million RNs in the United States, 25 percent no longer practice. Hospitals currently report about 100,000 nursing vacancies (Allen & Kraft, 1981).

Skyrocketing health care costs are forcing hospitals to take a close look at their expenditures. Health care costs rose 15.2 percent from 1979 to 1980, the biggest jump in 15 years, according to the Department of Health and Human Services; 60 percent of the increase was due to inflation (Dodge, 1981). With the present system of dealing with nursing personnel, most hospitals are only increasing their costs by hiring from medical pools.

Even the nurses who have stayed in the profession are spread out in other practice settings besides hospitals. Nurses today have private practices and run clinics in city and rural settings. New RNs can sign up for programs that let them travel to different hospitals around the country with travel expenses paid. Nurses can go abroad more easily, they can develop multi-part-time arrangements, and even occupy positions in organizations as wellness directors.

For the nurses who stay in hospitals, the clinical practice setting has changed dramatically. As recently as 1977, a typical medical-surgical floor in an urban hospital was not staffed with primary nurses and did not have patient classification, family centered care, or integrated progress notes. Today, many more hospitals have one or more of these, and the nurse has increased responsibility for the quality and quantity of patient care.

Coordination of Patient Care

The nurse's role has changed from that of mostly a direct caregiver to mainly a coordinator of the patient's care. With the rise in specialization in the medical system, a patient may have five or more different doctors. In a single day the nurse may have to coordinate the doctors, inhalation therapy, the x-ray and dietary departments, family visiting, direct patient care, and whatever tests are ordered. Nurses are seen as responsible for the smooth functioning of patient care. In many hospitals head nurses are called patient care coordinators.

Fortunately, there are also staff nurses giving direct patient care. We are beginning to see the return of primary nursing to the hospital scene and the development of clinical ladders for advancement. These patient care coordinators undergo a lot of stress in their position too. Rarely appreciated as the backbone of nursing, they begin to burn out. At whatever level you coordinate patient care, make sure you are doing your part to let those around you know you recognize and appreciate their contribution.

Increased Complexity of Care

The increased complexity of care calls for skills in the coordination of technical, psychological, and family-related dimensions of patient care. The coordination of complex care is seen most vividly in the jobs of ICU-CCU nurses. The complex work environment of ICU-CCU nurses has been described in many articles (Cassem & Hackett, 1975; Eisendrath & Dunkel, 1979; Oskins, 1979); the most descriptive summary is that by Gardner, Parzen, and Stewart (1980, pp. 103–104):

ICU-CCU: distracting noises emanate from the units' complex equipment and machinery . . confused patients in pain . . . insufficient space for nursing privacy . . . strenuous workload, which includes heavy lifting, monitoring numerous physical parameters, checking machinery, and meticulous recording of data . . . work pace highly unpredictable . . . present at all times . . . is the demand for quick and accurate decisions and faultless judgment . . . sight of acutely ill patients unconscious, deformed, and lying in blood and excretions . . . high mortality rate, presenting staff with repetitive losses and the necessity to reinvest physical and emotional energy in a new patient before they have adequately mourned the loss of a former patient to whom they had become attached emotionally . . .

frustration, anger, guilt and hopelessness may be felt in association with the patient who is dying, long-term, ventilator-dependent; elderly; antisocial; self-destructive; or drug and alcohol dependent . . . [Nurses are] frustrated by the patient's incomplete recovery on discharge from CCU, which deprives them of seeing the ultimate success of their strenuous efforts . . . interruptions because of the continual flow of hospital personnel through the ICU . . . physician-related problems—confronted with a critical, demanding physician who may leave them feeling insulted and humiliated or with a physician whose skills and judgment they mistrust and who leaves them feeling powerless and frustrated . . . [They are] frustrated at not being included in the planning of comprehensive patient care . . . [by being] asked to fulfill responsibilities belonging to the physician . . . lack of support and understanding from administration with issues such as staffing, compensatory time and need for time away from the unit . . . [The] expectation of faultless performance engenders feelings of great personal responsibility . . . [Nurses are] chronically plagued by fears of lacking adequate skill or knowledge . . . fear of harming patients by error of omission or commission in carrying out life-dependent tasks and they feel guilty when performing pain inflicting procedures such as suctioning, turning, coughing, and changing dressings . . . [They] feel frustrated when patients don't improve despite great efforts . . . measure self-worth by survival and improved patients therefore feel like failure when a patient deteriorates or dies.

All these physical, psychological, and mental stressors are part of working in the ICU-CCU unit.

Several authors, (Baily, Steffen, & Gnout, 1980; Huckabay & Jagla, 1979; Stehle, 1981; Vreeland & Ellis, 1969) divide the stressors into four major categories:

- Stressors that erupt from interpersonal communication problems.
- Stressors resulting from the nurses' need for an extensive knowledge base.
- Stressors present in an ICU environment.
- Stressors stemming from the rigors of patient care requirements.

These stressors are constantly present in the ICU. They illustrate the complexity of care in which some nurses are involved.

Burden of Nonnursing Responsibilities

A good nursing staff will perform their duties more or less satisfactorily under every disadvantage. But while doing so, their head will always try to improve their surroundings in such a way as to liberate them from subsidiary work, and to enable them to devote their time more exclusively to the care of the sick. This is, after all, the real purpose of their being there at all, not to act as lifts, water-carriers, beasts of burden, or steam engines—articles whose labour can be had at vastly less cost than that of educated human beings. (Florence Nightingale, 1867, quoted in Byrnes, 1982)

Unfortunately, over 100 years later, these nonnursing functions are still a major source of dissatisfaction in the nursing profession.

A source of such frustration is having to fulfill duties such as fetching a lunch tray because the dietary department forgot to change Mr. Jones from full liquid to a soft diet and they have no one to send the new tray. Another example is the evening nurse supervisor being responsible for dispensing drugs. Nonnursing duties are duties normally assumed by another department in most hospitals. Learning to "say no" to these duties or at least setting limits to these duties can relieve some of the stress nurses face.

Nurses need to stop covering up for the shortcomings of other services. For instance, perhaps the next time you have no laundry, call the director of this service and have him explain to Mr. Brown why he gets no sheets. Nurses need to clearly state to members of other disciplines that they have responsibilities. It is time for nurses to stop doing activities for which they get no fee and no recognition. Other services in hospitals do adjust to nursing departments setting limits.

Too often nurses forget that the hospital could not run without them. Nurses are an integral part of the hospital system in which they work. Any large system giving health care—from a public health system to a doctor's office—requires the skills of a nurse. If the nursing department or even a nursing floor is changed, the effect is felt throughout the whole medical organization.

The time has come for nurses to give up the three S's—subservience, self-sacrifice, and submissiveness (Maaksel, 1979). Nurses can no longer afford the time or energy to do nonnursing duties. It is too much of a burden to do all your work as a nurse and do someone else's job too. Paying a $15.00 an hour nurse to do a $5.00 an hour clerical or housekeeping task does not make sense in dollars either. For this reason administrators are now more ready to listen to nursing complaints. Utilize these dollar-and-sense statistics to convince your nursing department to take action.

Undervaluation of Profession

For hundreds of years nursing has allowed itself to be guided by administrators' and physicians' desires. Fortunately, today there is a somewhat dramatic shift in the attention paid to nurses. Hospital administrators, noting the shortage of nurses, have begun to encourage changes in policy to recruit and retain nurses. More money, benefits, and flexibility are available to nurses because administrators are now aware of their value.

Physicians are aware of nurses' value and either respect it or are threatened by it. Working in collaborative relationships with nurses, they see the nurses' increased expertise. The short-staffed conditions under which they work foster their empathy for the nurses' position. Some, however, because they need to be the authority, fear a loss of power, or for whatever other reason, treat nurses poorly. These physicians show little or no respect for nurses. They are critical in front of others. They operate from the position of telling the nurse the patient care orders, rather than planning them with the nurse. Nurses, like many women today, are no longer willing to tolerate being talked down to. Nurses, like other workers, want a say in the work process for which they are responsible.

Consumers are beginning to see nurses in a different light due to increased media coverage of the present nursing shortage and exposure to rural nurse practitioners and nurse specialists. Nursing has been the subject of articles in major national magazines ("Florence Nightingale," 1981; Johnson, 1981) and several network television shows. Patients leaving the hospitals can often do the best public relations job for nurses. Good patient care leaves a lasting impression in the mind of the public.

Raising the awareness of the consumer regarding the importance of nurses is useless unless nurses themselves appreciate their value in the health care system. The theme of the 1982 ANA convention was "Nursing: A Force of the Nation's Health."

Nurses themselves are often their worst enemy in regard to getting people to appreciate and reimburse them for their value. You could do a good deal for yourself and your profession by valuing yourself as a person and also as a nurse. Feeling proud of being a nurse will support you in your work environment. High self-esteem always makes it easier to cope with stress.

Nursing organizations and the National Commission on Nursing are searching for appropriate changes to improve the position of nurses in general. In this chapter you learn, as an individual nurse, how to diagnose, treat, and prevent work stress. Some solutions being developed on a national level are considered in Chapter 6.

IDENTIFYING AND REDUCING STRESS

Given all the stress-causing factors inherent in the role, individual nurses need to develop personal plans of action to assess their own level of job satisfaction. You need to determine the level of dissatisfaction that puts you at risk for burnout. The self-assessment instruments presented here are designed to help you assess some risk factors. The skills discussed can help you adjust to your working situation in order to maintain an acceptable level of stress.

Identifying your sources of dissatisfaction is the first step in creating a more satisfying work environment. Take time now to complete the survey presented in Table 5-1 so that you can approach the material presented later knowing your main areas of focus.

According to Herzburg's (1959) theories on job satisfaction, the areas you just examined fall into two categories: hygiene and motivating factors. Herzburg found that job dissatisfaction and job satisfaction factors were not the same. The job dissatisfaction aspects—the hygiene factors—are pay, working conditions, policies and administration, supervision, and security. These are the factors it is important to correct to help people be less dissatisfied with their work. Job satisfaction, however, is more than just not being dissatisfied. Factors such as advancement, recognition for accomplishment, achievement, challenging work, and increased responsibility are motivators. The presence of these motivators in your work environment fosters a satisfying work climate. List the factors that are lacking in your present position.

Once you have identified some of your sources of dissatisfaction, your next question is, "Is there anything I can do to change my present level of work dissatisfaction?" If the answer is "no," then you will need to put effort into using stress reduction techniques in your personal life. Increasing satisfaction in your personal life is not a long-term substitute for decreasing job dissatisfaction stress, but it can be a workable plan in the short run.

If the answer is "yes, there is something I can do," then approach the material presented here with that attitude in mind. Your physical environment is often thought of as the most difficult thing to change; however, nurses have been involved in the building of hospitals, the renovating of hospital units, and the painting of their units. White noise generators have been used to block out noise, and lighting has been changed after it was shown to be hazardous to patients and nursing personnel. These changes came about because nurses became involved in goal-directed planning and organizing.

At present, however, you need to focus on identifying sources of dissatisfaction and gathering ideas about how to improve the situation. The change process itself is postponed until later. In this chapter you are offered information that enables you to answer the question, "Is there anything I can do to change my present level of job dissatisfaction?" in the affirmative.

If your score on the context survey (Table 5-1) is over 45, it is important that you make a serious effort to find ways to improve your level of job satisfaction. The more dissatisfied you are at work, the higher is your stress level. You are either continually trying to rectify the situation or you take an "I don't care anymore" attitude and probably become

Table 5-1
CONTEXT SURVEY

1. How satisfied are you with the organization you work for compared with other organizations you know about?
2. How satisfied are you with your job—the kind of work you do?
3. How satisfied are you with your physical working conditions (heat, light, noise, etc.)?
4. How satisfied are you with the extent to which people you work with cooperate with one another?
5. How satisfied are you with the job your immediate supervisor is doing in managing his or her people responsibilities?
6. How satisfied are you with the job your immediate supervisor is doing in managing his or her functional responsibilities?
7. How satisfied are you with your pay, considering your duties and responsibilities?
8. How satisfied are you with your pay, considering what other organizations pay for similar types of work?
9. How satisfied are you with your advancement to better jobs since you started to work with your organization?
10. How satisfied are you with your opportunities to move into a better job in your organization?
11. How satisfied are you with the extent to which your present job makes use of your skills and abilities?
12. How satisfied are you with the level of mental ability requirements of your present job (problem solving, judgment, technical knowledge, etc.)?
13. How satisfied are you with the level of average time demands of your present job (hours worked)?
14. Now, considering everything, how would you rate your overall feelings about your employment situation at the present time?
15. If you have your way, will you be working for your present organization five years from now?*

How to score
Assign one number to each question according to the following scale:

    1 = Very satisfied
    2 = Satisfied
    3 = Neutral
    4 = Dissatisfied
    5 = Very dissatisfied

It is important that you answer every question.
*For this question, score as follows:

    1 = Certainly
    2 = Probably
    3 = I am not at all sure
    4 = Probably not

5 = Certainly not

6 = I will be retired in five years

Total scores can range from 14 to 75. Scores of 45 or more may suggest that the overall context of your work is less than satisfactory. You should also evaluate the specific items in the survey that you rated negatively. Stop and think about those areas of dissatisfaction. List the primary areas that are sources of stress for you. Do these create low job dissatisfcation for you? Your level of stress and your level of job satisfaction are integrally connected.

depressed. In fact, either approach will lead to burnout. A dissatisfying work environment makes it hard to take care of others and very difficult to take care of yourself.

An increasingly negative attitude toward work needs quick attention, for your negativity will also begin to affect your feelings toward yourself. You will begin to focus on your limitations and mistakes and develop a low self-esteem. If you are not only dissatisfied with your work, but with your personal life too, you must launch an immediate attack to improve your situation. If you do not treat the signs of burnout, you will probably end up being treated for depression or some physical illness.

The solution often is not quitting your job; "the grass is greener" route has misled many disappointed nurses. Before you quit, at least read Chapter 8 and attempt to reduce the stress at your current job. Changing yourself and rallying support for work changes always seem more difficult than they actually are.

For instance, nurses can rally support to change a major issue leading to dissatisfaction—nonnursing duties. In the context survey (Table 5-1) the question of the extent to which your job makes use of your abilities (no. 11) focuses on the issue of nonnursing duties. If you spend your time emptying trash, making unoccupied beds, stamping charts, filling out x-ray requests, and serving meal trays, you are likely not to have answered "satisfied" to the question 11.

Nonnursing duties generally fall into five categories: housekeeping, clerical, transportation, dietary, and miscellaneous (Byrnes, 1982). Often nurses are asked to assume other departments' responsibilities on evenings, nights, and weekends—the same time nursing manpower is reduced. Some nurses have commented that they average one hour a day or more doing tasks such as filling out reports that do not require nursing knowledge, cleaning up after physicians, following up on supplies not delivered, etc. These nonnursing tasks inflate the shortage and raise the stress level of nurses.

What can you do? First determine precisely what nonnursing functions you are performing. Consulting a list of these functions (Byrnes, 1982, p. 1097) could help you get focused. As an educator or administrator you would add other items to this list. Some faculty are expected to type their own tests!

Once you have your list of nonnursing duties, make recommendations that specifically reflect the issues. For instance, the housekeeping staff empties trash on day shift, however, by the end of evening shift the nurse is required to empty trash cans. Recommend that one housekeeper could cover several units on evenings and nights, with the bulk of the work still done on days. That person could also mop up the spills that occur on evenings and nights. Nonnursing clerical duties frequently listed are answering telephones, forwarding charts, ordering supplies, filling out lab slips and x-ray requests, calling labs and x-ray departments for results, making clinic appointments, checking patients' clothing and valuables, and charting temperatures and blood work (Byrnes, 1982). You could recommend assigning a ward clerk to each unit for each shift, developing a training course for the ward clerks, or hiring a unit manager for each unit. All of these would be cost-effective ways to handle clerical duties.

There are several other variables that contribute to your job satisfaction. By focusing specifically on a few, you could turn the tide of your disappointment in your present job or even in nursing in general. The variables listed in various sources are best illustrated by the eight principal variables in overall job satisfaction identified by Albrecht (1979). Each of these variables is briefly described below. Rate each one on a scale of 1–5: 5 means mostly satisfied, 3 means sometimes satisfied, and 1 means rarely satisfied. For example, if you are rarely satisfied with your workload you would rate it 1.

JOB SATISFACTION TEST

- *Workload.* Believe it or not, some nurses complain of too little work and feel bored! Most of you are on the opposite end of the continuum, complaining of overload. Role overload, whether quantitative or qualitative, decreases the quality of your work life. Short staffing is common across the country. If this is not a problem for you, count your blessings.
- *Physical variables.* Temperature, humidity, little or no light, noise, and chemicals are all factors affecting your physical environment. How many nurses would like to see a window in their unit or office? Also include here crowding and having to do fatiguing tasks.

- *Job status.* A low or negative social status creates psychological discomfort. Nurses have increased their status through using different titles, such as "clinical care coordinator" instead of "head nurse." Your status may be recognized by the size and location of your office or the courses you are selected to teach.
- *Accountability.* This is the extent? to which important outcomes depend on your performance in relation to the amount of control you have over the results. If you are repeatedly held responsible for situations in which you have little control, if you are involved in a considerable amount of "busy work" (meaningless work), or you get no useful feedback on task effectiveness, this aspect of your work is not satisfactory.
- *Task variety.* The continuum goes from deadly dull, monotonous, repetitive, to unpredictable, unprogramed, always changing. Either end is accompanied by frustration and no sense of real accomplishment. Is your task variety balanced so that you are satisfied with this variable?
- *Human contact.* Occasionally administrators and/or nurses complain about too little human contact. However, most nurses have desert island fantasies by the end of the day because they are so stimulated by people overload. Nurses sometimes call this being "peopled-out." Do you want more or less human contact, or are you satisfied?
- *Physical challenge.* How much dexterity, physical skill or strength, endurance, or physical mobility do you need on your job? If you are a highly physical person and your job has little activity you are likely to experience some degree of frustration. Talking and operating a ballpoint pen may be the only physical challenge some administrators and professors get. Perhaps you are not a physical person and this little activity is satisfying for you at work. Be kind to your body and moderately exercise after work, especially if your job is sedentary.
- *Mental challenge.* People perform better if they use their cognitive skills to some degree. These skills include observing, recognizing, memorizing, monitoring, comparing, evaluating, deciding, and reasoning. If you are underchallenged you probably feel frustrated and experience a desire to escape to something more stimulating for your mind. If you are overloaded with mental challenges you probably experience inadequacy in coping with them.

Which of these eight factors, along with pay and benefits, do you think might have the most impact on your worklife? The answer to this question lies in the variables you listed as being the least satisfactory. Which variables did you rate 1 or 2? List two of the variables that have the most impact your work life. In the next section, titled Understanding

Your System, there is an outline of a process you can use to begin to take action on these.

Whatever variables you decided were most significant, changing them is initially going to be more difficult than adapting yourself to them; this is the reason people usually initially try to adapt their behavior to the situation they are in. Trying to get your supervisor to treat you as a thinking adult or trying to get Mary to arrive on time may seem impossible. We take the easier road because to choose the other path would create *conflict*.

Women have been enculturated to avoid upsetting anyone with their wants. (I find even male nurses are not immune to this problem.) Conflict is to be avoided: for example, avoid getting people angry by telling them you want them to follow the rules and be on time. It is likely that changing these variables to be more satisfying will involve conflict situations. Conflict resolution skills are discussed later in this chapter.

The personality pattern of adapting to a situation by trying to change yourself to fit in creates a loss of work self-esteem. You begin to question not only the other's competence, but also your own. You may not see the direct connection between work overload or high accountability and seeing yourself as inefficient and ineffective. There is a connection between your identified work dissatisfaction variables and the anxiety, depression, or physical signs you are experiencing.

The price you pay for adapting to a situation can be high. Before you say "I quit," try relating to your job from an assertive position of risking conflict to resolve your dissatisfaction variables. It may be as simple as switching shifts, your unit, or your specialty area. You know what work factors need to be changed. You will begin to learn how to change them by reading this book. Armed with this information and a little courage and support from your friends and colleagues, you can begin to take action to increase your level of work satisfaction.

If you do not take care of yourself you will reach the third stage of burnout. In this stage you will be angry and resentful of the patients—the very people you wanted to help—and the meaning of your work will be lost. Absence of meaning in one's work leads to feeling, "It is not worth it. I don't feel proud of being a nurse. What I do for these patients is insignificant."

You have heard these statements and others like them. The question is, what system takes a bright, energetic, caring person and turns him or her into someone who is depressed, resentful, and uncaring? The medical and nursing systems are finally changing because nurses refuse to adapt, and adapt, and end up burned out. Only you, via personal and professional action, can turn the tide.

UNDERSTANDING YOUR SYSTEM

Understanding your system, whether it is a hospital, public health agency, or nursing school, requires that you learn some basic facts about the health care system (Kraegal, 1980; Magula, 1982). Health care organizations are not the same as business and industrial organizations. In the health care business the goal of the personnel is to deliver a high-quality service, whereas in the business world the goal is to make money by delivering a service or selling a product.

One of the major problems in health care is that the two different viewpoints of service and money operate within the same organization. Nurses and other health care personnel believe the goal of the organization is to deliver high-quality service to the patient. The administration, almost by definition, needs to be concerned with money. The other personnel are often in conflict with the administration that runs the place because the administration has the political and financial power. However, the recent emergence of for-profit hospitals is showing that making money and delivering quality care do not need to be mutually exclusive endeavors.

The first two points to remember about changing a system are (1) understand that this conflict always exists, and (2) find out who on the administrative level can be counted on to rally for the creation of a more satisfying work climate for nurses. Know who supports your goal of quality patient care before you begin your tactical approach. They should possess qualities of assertiveness and a willingness to stand up for what they value and believe (not the kind of standing up where they win the battle and lose the war, but the kind where their belief is powered by assertive, politically wise behavior—knowing when and where not to be assertive is one aspect of being politically wise.)

Like it or not, politics is here to stay. In any organization that uses power to control its people, volleying for control of the resources will be the main attraction in the political arena. You, as nurses, are one of the resources they are trying to control. You need to take control or they will take control of you.

Your supporters have varying degrees of leadership skills—what is important is that they know when to lead and when to follow. A plaque on the desk of an executive in a company for which I consulted read, "Lead, follow, or get out of the way." This states the issue succinctly.

The final quality of those you can count on is that they *care*. They care about people, care about nursing as a profession, and care about themselves. Nurses are beginning to realize that being an effective nurse means better patient care. In order to be effective they need to give up their submissive role and risk conflict.

The first step in bringing someone to your way of thinking is to know specifically what you want to accomplish (goal). You would never think of heading up the football field without a clear purpose in mind. If you want to get a salary increase for your nursing managerial responsibilities, justify the cost effectiveness of all RN staff, or stress the importance of less leniency in assessing the clinical competence of your students, the first step is to clearly define that goal.

The second step is to know what the others think of your goal. Know what their first negative response would be, the second, third, and so on. Your plan of action has to have an approach to deal with each of these reactions. The more strongly they are likely to resist the change, the more homework you need to do on facts and the more you need support in numbers.

Banding together your forces is a key strategy in changing a work environment. You, as a nurse, need support to make most of the changes you need in your work environment. Please remember—if you decide to try single-handedly to change the system that is creating your work stress, you are probably tackling a symptom of the problem, rather than a cause. (Or you need to sit and examine your heroine needs!) Most heroes go unnoticed because they fail.

Knowing your goal and the steps to accomplish this goal, as well as others' probable reactions will lead you to develop a rational, flexible, and farsighted plan. Treating symptoms of work stress has not worked for nursing. Your time is better spent with a plan that involves alleviation of problems now and in the future. Understanding the dynamics of your large organizational system can help you plan changes even on your individual role level. Politics and the issues of support, loyalty, and leadership operate on each work level. Just these three issues profoundly affect your role delineation.

CLARIFYING YOUR ROLE: ROLE CONFLICT AND ROLE AMBIGUITY

Clarification of certain aspects of your role as a nurse can reduce work stress. Role conflict and role ambiguity are two role definition and delineation problems cited frequently in the stress literature. Understanding the cause and developing coping strategies for each will help reduce the stress produced by conflict and uncertainty.

Role conflict is the experience of being pulled in several directions by people with different expectations of how you should behave as a nurse. These differences may concern what your priorities of patient care should be, how you dress, or how you should teach psychiatric nursing. Management may expect you to make their paperwork a priority, while your staff wants you to help them with their busy clinical work. You may feel your priority is emotional patient care and yet have a number of patients to care for physically. In the first example the role conflict is triggered by direct external demands, in the latter, the role conflict is internal.

Kahn and Rosenthal (1964) have identified four types of role conflicts. How many of these are part of your present position conflicts?

ROLE CONFLICT TEST

- Inconsistent demands from another individual (e.g., manager encourages your ideas then discredits them repeatedly in management meetings).
- Incompatible demands on you from two or more organization members (e.g., unit is short staffed, so that even though you are the manager of the unit, i.e., head nurse, you are also expected to fill in clinically).
- Pressures to act in one way in a formal position in the organization, and to act in another as a member of an informal network in the organization (e.g., as professor you are expected to maintain a certain degree of distance to remain objective, and as the sophomore class leader you are expected to be friendly and supportive of class).
- Behaviors demanded by organization members in conflict with your personal values or morals (e.g., demands to ignore patient safety regulations).

If you find yourself in two or more of these conflicts, then you are probably experiencing a significant amount of frustration and stress. First, make a list of the conflicts you face in your work climate, then prioritize your list. You may choose to begin action on one of them before you have completed reading this book.

First check to see if the stress is being internally generated or if the conflict comes from external demands. How many times have you worried about a problem when no problem existed? If you repeatedly create internal conflict, then go back and reread the section on perfectionism in Chapter 3.

If the conflict is external, then you need to sit down separately with each person with a conflicting expectation. You may need to sit down with them together also. If your first response was that it would not work for you, think again. Most people, when approached in a responsible, rational way, will respond in the same way. Mustering the courage to do it usually is the problem. Confronting the potential conflict and ending up with the other person not liking you is a scary thing to do. Realize that when you avoid your conflict problems, you end up paying a high price—that of work stress.

Role ambiguity is similar to role conflict in that the individual experiences stress due to conflict, however, in this case the conflicts result from unclear responsibilities. There is inadequate information about what work you should cover, the limits on your work behavior in the role, and other people's expectations of how your role fits with their roles. For example, a new head nurse is experiencing stress because she is given no guidelines in her new job in the outpatient department because she has been with the organization for ten years working in the emergency room. Stress comes from the feeling of uncertainty, the lack of defining structure.

Lyons (1971) showed that perceived role ambiguity among RNs is related to turnover. Both Kahn et al., (1964) and Lyons (1971) found that the need for clarity appeared to moderate the relationship between role ambiguity and job-related tension. In other words, an individual with a high need for structure would have more tension in an ambiguous job.

Three possible solutions to role ambiguity exist. One is to overwork, and another is withdraw from work. The third involves using your courage and your skills to get a clear role delineation with all relevant parties.

To check whether you use overwork as a solution, answer the questions in Table 5-2 with either a "yes" or a "no" and evaluate your answers at the end of the questionnaire.

If your answers frequently matched those given at the end of the table, then you can consider yourself a workaholic. Depending on who you talk with, you will get different advice concerning this diagnosis. Machlowitz (1980) points out that workaholics are often happy people. They are intense and energetic; they wake up and cannot wait to get going. Machlowitz interviewed hundreds of work addicts and found that most were happy because they were doing what they enjoyed—working. The people who work for or live with workaholics often suffer, however (Lavandero, 1981). Adjusting to the frantic schedule of a workaholic is not easy and rarely rewarding. Many workaholics are married to their work.

Friedman and Rosenman (1974) state that not all workaholics have Type A personalities. Those that are Type A are likely to become heart attack victims because they adopt a destructive behavior pattern in which they respond to all kinds of stress by attempting to work even harder. If you registered high on the Type A quiz (Table 3-5) and also registered as a workaholic (Table 5-2) then you might try some of these ways to detach from excessive work centeredness: reading novels or poetry, going to the movies, dancing, hiking or backpacking, watching sunsets, spending time with friends, traveling, or reconnecting with a spiritual tradition.

Table 5-2.
ARE YOU A WORKAHOLIC?

1. Do you seem to communicate better with your secretary (co-workers) than with your spouse (or best friend)?
2. Are you always punctual for appointments?
3. Are you better able to relax on Saturdays than on Sunday afternoons?
4. Are you more comfortable when you are productive than idle?
5. Do you carefully organize your hobbies?
6. Are you usually much annoyed when your spouse (or friend) keeps you waiting?
7. When you play golf is it mainly with business associates? (Are most recreational activities with work associates?)
8. Does your spouse (or friend) think of you as an easygoing person?
9. If you play tennis do you occasionally see (or want to see) your boss's face on the ball before a smash?
10. Do you tend to substitute your work for interpersonal contacts; that is, is work sometimes a way of avoiding close relationships?
11. Even under pressure, do you usually take the extra time to make sure you have *all* the facts before making a decision?
12. Do you usually plan every step of the itinerary of a trip in advance and tend to become uncomfortable if plans go awry?
13. Do you enjoy small talk at a reception or cocktail party?
14. Are most of your friends in the same line of work?
15. Do you take work to bed with you when you are home sick?
16. Is most of your reading work related?
17. Do you work late more frequently than your peers?
18. Do you talk "shop" over cocktails on social occasions?
19. Do you wake up in the night worrying about business problems?
20. Do your dreams tend to center on work-related conflicts?
21. Do you play as hard as you work?

Answers

1. Yes	8. No	15. Yes
2. Yes	9. Yes	16. Yes
3. Yes	10. Yes	17. Yes
4. Yes	11. Yes	18. Yes
5. Yes	12. Yes	19. Yes
6. Yes	13. No	20. Yes
7. Yes	14. Yes	21. Yes

The overwork solution is usually seen in the overresponsible individual. Controlling and rescuing types usually take this approach. These are the people who, instead of clarifying the arithmetic homework assignment in grade school, did all the problems! This solution leads to physical burnout, for the body cannot take all the extra work.

The person who withdraws usually flees from the work with comments such as, "It is not my responsibility." This attitude develops because unresolved, frustrating experiences lead to defeat. Instead of controlling by behaving like the overworker, these nurses control by withholding their help. They may underwork not only out of anger at the ambiguous situation, but also because they are afraid that they will make a mistake because the work overload has affected their thinking. Underworkers withdraw in order to cope. They stop working because to do the job creates more psychic pain than not doing it. If people do the best they can and then someone repeatedly gives them no credit and finds only their mistakes, they are likely to head for the underwork side of burnout.

Where does your responsibility begin and end? This question is important to answer. The answer will change over the course of your career, but whatever job you have, know your responsibilities. Knowing your job description, working according to it, and being paid fairly for it will reduce considerable stress. Take time to list two actions you can take to reduce role conflict and/or role ambiguity. List two concrete actions you could do to reduce the stress of unclear role delineation.

SKILLS TO DECREASE WORK STRESS

Setting limits on your role can involve conflict situations. Probably more than any other, the assertive techniques of "saying no" and setting limits are needed to regulate your work environment. They are ways to take control of your time management at work. These skills, plus conflict resolution and collaborative problem solving, are necessary to change your work to make it more satisfying.

Saying No

"Saying no" is a skill because it involves an empathetic understanding of the other person's position, as well as assertive communication skills. "No" can be said in an assertive, nonrebellious, tactful way.

Many times it feels uncomfortable to say "no," and almost 100 percent of the time we do not like hearing "no." "No" means we do not get "our way" and we usually want our way. Do you remember in your developmental psychology courses the stress placed on the importance of saying appropriate "no's" in raising children? Children need limits; therefore, adults need to say "no." You may be thinking "I did not like 'no' as a child and I do not like it much more now." The only difference betwen a two-year-old's response and yours, as an adult nurse, is that you have been socialized into believing that throwing a temper tantrum is selfish, rude, and certain to create posttantrum embarrassment. You are more civilized; you swallow your response to the "no" and instead create ulcers or depression.

The response you get to saying no depends on how you say it (assertive, aggressive, or passive aggressive) and when you say it. Remember the tactful political nature you are developing. Always check yourself with, "Is saying 'yes/no' in my best interests?" Then ask yourself about others' needs. Too often you do the latter first and forget the former question. Instead of internally creating the feelings of being unappreciated, taken advantage of, or resentful, say no and feel self-respect.

You may hurt someone's feelings with an assertive 'no'; the hurt will heal. Passive-aggressive (talking behind their backs) or aggressive (sarcastic, abusive language) substitutes cut deeply into people and the cut heals very slowly. Empathetic assertion will accomplish saying no and support your self-respect as well as the other's self-respect.

Saying no is important in setting limits. However, saying yes can also define your limits. For instance, you may say no to being on a committee for designing a patient classification system, but say yes to committees to improve the working relationships between hospital departments. In this way you are defining your own limits.

Expanding your limits by venturing out of your comfort zone for a challenging task or an adventure has to bring some rewards. Without some monetary, verbal, or intrinsic rewards the task will seem burdensome. In setting your limits, allow for sufficient stability and risk. This requires continual monitoring of your personal and professional needs.

When you become unclear about your needs or do not set your life up to meet your needs, you experience psychic conflict. Inner conflict is your mind's way of telling you that you need to say no to one choice and say yes to another. Your choice needs to be based on your needs and the requirements of the situation.

Conflict arises between you and someone else for the same reason. If your needs are in conflict you experience stress. If your needs conflict with others' needs then you are likely to experience some degree of stress. Being able to resolve conflicts with others is an important stress-reducing skill.

Conflict Resolution

In order to resolve a conflict, both parties need to recognize its source. Many times the issue that triggered the conflict is not the source. Careful examination with clear communication is necessary to identify the source.

After you understand the source of the conflict, the second step is to utilize acceptable strategies to solve the conflict. Different methods for resolving conflict are available; the best choice depends upon the source of the conflict and the importance of the issue.

Conflicts between individuals stem from the dynamic interplay of individual as well as organizational factors. Individual characteristics such as defensiveness, authoritarianism, aggressiveness, stress from overloading, and prejudice can lead to interaction patterns of competition and domination (Filley, 1975). Conflict is more likely in rigid, autocratic organizations according to Likert and Likert (1976). They suggest that management practices that encourage teamwork, participative decision making, and two-way communication minimize conflict.

Whatever the source of conflict, the emotions involved in the situation need to be dealt with first. When your adrenalin is flowing you are prepared for fighting, not for problem solving. To reach the point of rational problem solving, either party needs to decide to bring the situation under control. Staying away from putdowns, experiencing the argument of the other, and stating your views and feelings are all part of the listening and asserting approach.

How the conflict is resolved depends mostly on the persons involved in the conflict. We each have our favorite way. Many people have a way based not upon logic, but upon habit. Hart (1981) has identified the five most common methods; they are described in Table 5-3. Their appropriateness depends upon the issues involved in the conflict.

Collaborative Problem Solving

Each of these methods involves the idea of win/lose. Only collaboration results in a win/win result. Gordon and Burch (1974) describe a process for the resolution of interpersonal problems. The parties involved join together to find an acceptable solution for both. This method entails redefining the problem, discovering novel alternatives, and focusing on overlapping interests. The six-step process is outlined in Table 5-4 (Bolton, 1979). For further information, see Gordon (1977) and Gordon and Burch (1974).

An example of this method of collaborative problem solving was seen in a hospital that decided to further improve the skills of its management level staff in running meetings. A consultant acted as a facilitator as the group defined the problem. The problem was not just the running of meetings, but also increasing the cohesiveness of the staff members so that they would feel freer to express themselves in meetings. In brainstorming, the group came up with 15 different ideas. Task forces were formed to work on the six major issues. A format for reporting back was decided upon and the method of evaluation was formulated. Follow-up meetings were to be held at monthly intervals.

The same process can work between two individuals who are in conflict. For example, a head nurse came to her boss with her resignation. She explained she could no longer work 7–3 because her husband and she were getting a divorce and he would no longer be able to care for the children during the day. She explained that her mother could care for them from 9 until 5 and her husband could care for them after 5

When the problem was defined in terms of needs rather than solutions, the need was clearly for responsible caretaking of the children. Her quitting her job was the result of defining the problem in terms of solution. During brainstorming of options, the idea of her working 9–5 was mentioned. When all the choices were considered, this one was selected on a trial basis. The further outcome of this study was that flexible hours were instituted for all head nurses after a three-month trial with this nurse.

CHOOSING THE BEST CAREER PATH

One of the best ways to prevent work stress is to find the right job for yourself. When you are feeling satisfied and enjoy your job, then your work stress will be at a comfortable level. You will see the stress as challenging and as part of an exciting job. Choosing your best career path is therefore the key.

To prevent work stress symptoms you need to keep a watchful eye on your level of nervous tension. Saying no is a stress prevention skill to reduce tension. You need to realize how often you feel, "This job is driving me crazy . . . driving me to drink . . . keeping me awake at night . . . giving me ulcers . . ." whatever is your symptom of tension. Unheeded, these feelings can result in physical, psychological, and behavioral stress symptoms. Making sure you are in a good job for you helps prevent these work stress symptoms. A brief lesson on choosing a career path or job follows.

To choose a career you have to know your work values, your interests, and your skills. You then mix and match these until you come up with the best choice combining all three. As you grow to understand

Table 5-3
FIVE BASIC METHODS FOR RESOLVING CONFLICT

Method	What Happens When Used	When Appropriate to Use	When Inappropriate to Use
Denial or withdrawal	Person tries to solve problem by denying its existence. Results in win/lose.	Issue is relatively unimportant and timing is wrong; cooling off period is needed; short-term use.	Issue is important; issue will not disappear, but build.
Suppression or smoothing over	Differences are played down; surface harmony exists. Results in win/lose in forms of resentment, defensiveness, and possibly sabotage if issue remains suppressed.	Same as above; also, preservation of relationship is more important than the issue at the moment.	Evasion of an important issue; others are ready and willing to deal with issue.
Power or dominance	One's authority, position, majority rule, or a persuasive minority settles the conflict. Results in win/lose if the dominated party sees no hope for self.	Power comes with position of authority; this method has been agreed upon.	Losers have no way to express needs; could result in future disruptions.

Compromise or negotiation	Each party gives up something in order to meet midway. Results in win/lose if "middle of the road" position ignores the real diversity of the issue.	Both parties have enough leeway to give; resources are limited; win/lose stance is undesirable.	Solution is too watered down to be effective.
Collaboration	Abilities, values, and expertise of all are recognized; each person's position is clear, but emphasis is on group solution. Results in win/win for all.	Time is available to complete the process; parties are committed and trained in use of process.	The proper conditions of time, abilities, and commitment are not present.

Reprinted from *Learning From Conflict: A Handbook for Trainers*, by Lois B. Hart, copyright © 1981, by permission of Addison-Wesley Publishing Co., Reading, Mass.

Table 5-4
COLLABORATIVE PROBLEM-SOLVING METHOD

I.   *Define the problem in terms of needs, not solutions.*
     A. Find out why the person wants the solution he or she initially proposed; understand the advantages that solution has for that person. "What do you want to achieve by working only day shift?" "What's in it for you to refuse the test?"
     B. Change perception from win/lose to win/win orientation by changing from false and limited perception of the nature of the problem.
         1. "I need to (statement of goals, not solution)."
         2. Assert your own needs, listen reflectively until you understand the other person's needs, and then state both sets of needs in a one-sentence summary of the problem.
         3. "A problem well defined is half-solved."

II. *Brainstorm possible solutions.*
     A. Rapidly generate and list solution ideas without clarification and without evaluation of their merits.
     B. Try for quantity, not quality.
     C. Basic guidelines:
         1. Do not evaluate: evaluation thwarts creativity and makes people defensive.
         2. Do not clarify or seek clarification; it interferes with rapid creative solutions.
         3. Go for zany ideas; they act as relaxants and foster creativity.
         4. Expand each other's ideas.
         5. List every idea; do not censor.
         6. Avoid attaching people's names to the ideas they suggest or listing each person's contribution separately; concentrate on the group effort.

III. *Select the solution (or combination of solutions) that will best meet both parties' needs.*
     A. Make clarification as succinct as possible.
     B. Guidelines for evaluation:
         1. Ask what proposed alternatives are favored for the solution.
         2. State which alternatives look best to you.
         3. See which choices coincide.
         4. Jointly decide on one or more of the alternatives.
     C. Be sure the other person is satisfied with the solution.
     D. Try to reach a consensus—a sense of the meeting, a willingness to accept the group's decision.
     E. Foresee the possible consequences of that solution.

IV. *Plan who will do what and where*
     A. Clarify nitty-gritty of how solution is to be implemented.
     B. Methods to be used are also important.
     C. Write out the agreement reached.

V.   *Implement the plan: each person does his or her part in agreed-upon steps.*

VI. *Evaluate the problem-solving process and, at a later date, how well the solution turned out.*

Adapted from Bolton, R. *People skills.* Englewood Cliffs, NJ: Prentice-Hall, 1979.

these three aspects of yourself you will begin to see the best career direction for you. The same principles apply each time you look for a different job.

Career development, especially for nurses interested in bedside care, was a principal topic of discussion at the public hearings conducted by the National Commission on Nursing in February and March of 1981 (American Hospital Association, 1981). The ANA Commission on Nursing Services indicated that incentives, such as a salary system recognizing clinical achievement, could help reduce nurse turnover in hospitals. Nurses need a choice of potential tracks for advancement other than management and education.

Work Values

Before you decide which career track to pursue, reevaluate your most important work values using Table 5-5, which lists a wide variety of satisfactions that people obtain from their jobs. Do the exercise described at the end of the table. Now, from the list of 4's, choose the five values most important to you today and list them. Then give these values some thought and answer these questions: (1) Can I incorporate them into my present job? (2) Which do I need to keep in mind as I consider career alternatives?

Now that you are aware of what values are most important to you, begin to think of ways of incorporating them into your present work situation. If incorporating them seems infeasible, then you need to explore a different career path in nursing. Too often nurses, instead of exploring nursing options, allow themselves to burn out in their present position and then leave nursing. Use your values as guideposts; however, before you make your choice, also do the interest and skill assessments presented in Figure 5-1 and Table 5-6.

Interest Inventory

The following exercise adapted from Simon, Howe, and Kirschenbaum (1972), is designed to help you identify your interests, the things that you have enjoyed doing in your working life or think you would enjoy.

Following a format such as that presented in Figure 5-1, list the things you really like to do. Try to list at least 20. Include anything that makes you feel good and gives you satisfaction. These can be simple things, such as giving a backrub to a patient, hiring new nurses' aides, or

Table 5-5
WORK VALUES

Help society: Do something to contribute to the betterment of the world I live in.
Help others: Be involved in helping other people in a direct way, either individually or in small groups.
Public contact: Have a lot of day-to-day contact with people.
Work with others: Have close working relationships with a group; work as a team toward common goals.
Affiliation: Be recognized as a member of a particular organization.
Friendships: Develop close personal relationships with people as a result of my work activities.
Competition: Engage in activities that pit my abilities against others' where there are clear win-and-lose outcomes.
Make decisions: Have the power to decide courses of action, policies, etc.
Work under pressure: Work in situations where time pressure is prevalent and/or the quality of my work is judged critically by supervisors, customers, or others.
Power and authority: Control the work activities or (partially) the destinies of other people.
Influence people: Be in a position to change attitudes or opinions of other people.
Work alone: Do projects by myself, without any significant amount of contact with others.
Knowledge: Engage in the pursuit of knowledge, trust, and understanding.
Orderliness of environment: Work in a consistently orderly environment, where everything has its place and things are not changed often.
Undemanding: Have work duties that demand very little energy or involvement.
Personal growth and development: Engage in work that offers me an opportunity to grow as a person.
Intellectual status: Be regarded as a person of high intellectual prowess or as one who is an acknowledged "expert" in a given field.
Artistic creativity: Engage in creative work in any of several art forms.
Creativity (general): Create new ideas, programs, organizational structures, or anything else not following a format previously developed by others.
Aesthetics: Be involved in studying or appreciating the beauty of things, ideas, etc.
Supervision: Have a job in which I am directly responsible for the work done by others.
Change and variety: Have work responsibilities that frequently change in their content and setting.
Precision work: Work in situations where there is very little tolerance for error.
Stability: Have work routine and job duties that are largely predictable and not likely to change over a long period of time.
Security: Be assured of keeping my job and a reasonable financial reward.
Necessity: Feel that what I do is necessary for the survival or welfare of others.
Fast pace: Work in circumstances where there is a high pace of activity, work must be done rapidly.

Recognition: Be recognized for the quality of my work in some visible or public way.

Excitement: Experience a high degree of (or frequent) excitement in the course of my work.

Adventure: Have work duties that involve frequent risk taking.

Profit, gain: Have a strong likelihood of accumulating large amounts of money or other material gain.

Independence: Be able to determine the nature of my work without significant direction from others; not have to do what others tell me to.

Moral fulfillment: Feel that my work is contributing significantly to a set of moral standards that I feel are very important.

Location: Find a place to live (town, geographical area) that is conducive to my lifestyle and affords me the opportunity to do the things I enjoy most.

Community: Live in a town or city where I can get involved in community affairs.

Physical work environment: Work in a place that is pleasing to me aesthetically, is beautiful to me.

Fun: Work in a situation in which I am free to be spontaneous, playful, humorous, exuberant.

Uniqueness: Feel that the work I do is unique, novel, different from others' in some way.

Expertise: Be respected and sought after for my knowledge and expertise in a given area.

Physical challenge: Have a job that makes physical demands that I would find rewarding.

Time freedom: Have work responsibilities that I can work at according to my own time schedule; no specific working hours required.

High earnings anticipated: Monetary rewards would be such that I am able to purchase those things I consider essential and the luxuries of life I wish.

Status: Have a position that commands the respect of my friends, family, and community.

Advancement: The opportunity to work hard and make rapid career advancement.

Challenging problems: The position does not have to be "essential to the survival of the human race," but it should provide challenging problems to solve and the avoidance of continual routine.

Creative expression: Opportunity to express in writing or verbally my ideas, reactions, and observations concerning my job and how I might improve it.

Job tranquility: To avoid pressure and "the rat race."

Work on frontiers of knowledge: (a) Be involved in hard science or human research. (b) Work in a company that is considered one of the best in the business and strive for better product advances.

Exercise competence: An opportunity to involve myself in those areas in which I feel I have talents above the average person.

Productive: Produce tangibles, things that I can see and touch.

(continued)

Table 5-5 *(continued)*

How to score

Rate the degree of importance that you would assign to each of the above items using the following scale:

  1 = Not important at all
  2 = Not very but somewhat important
  3 = Reasonably important
  4 = Very important in my choice of career

Make separate lists of all those you chose as "1," "2," "3," and "4." Do you notice any patterns? Would you have rated them differently ten years ago? Five years ago? One year ago?

Reprinted from Figler, H. E. *Path: A career workbook for liberal arts students.* Cranston, R.I.: Carroll Press, 1979. With permission.

giving a positive evaluation to a student. They may be more difficult, such as preparing and presenting a lecture on your specialty area, firing a chronic problem staff member, or helping a family cope with the effects of disability in their aging mother. To get ideas, think of your day, people you work with, the roles you play. Think about work activities that you would like to do more often.

After you have completed your list, code these items in the columns to the right, following the key below the figure. Now go over your list. Choose the ten things you love to do the most and mark them with an asterisk in column 9. This interest inventory can act to guide you in identifying the things you most like to do in your work. Once you have identified those work aspects the next step is to see if you could incorporate more of them into your present position. If not, then you need to begin thinking about what nursing unit or nursing specialty could foster your interests.

Assessing Skills

If you are thinking about changing jobs you need to assess your current skills and decide what new skills you are interested in learning. Table 5-6 will help you in your assessment of these skills. To begin your own nursing skills inventory, list ten or more of your specialty *clinical skills*. Next, consider the *management skills* enumerated in Table 5-6, and make a list of those skills you feel comfortable in performing. Form another list of those you would like to learn. Repeat this for the *education skills*. Now, go back over your lists and for each group, circle the three skills that are most important to you.

Developing new skills is also to be considered. You may choose a

INTEREST INVENTORY									
My Interests: What I Enjoy Doing	P M S	TR	C	E	A	A O	PR	V	*
1.									
2.									
3.									
4.									
5.									
6.									
7.									
8.									
9.									
10.									
11.									
12.									
13.									
14.									
15.									
16.									
17.									
18.									
19.									
20.									

FIGURE 5-1. Interest inventory Key:

Column 1: Put a *P, M, S,* or a combination of the three, next to each item, depending on whether you use *physical, mental,* or *social skills.*

Column 2: Put a *TR* next to those that are usually regarded as part of a traditionally male or female role.

Column 3: Put a *C* next to those that are of a clinical nature.

Column 4: Put an *E* next to those that involve you acting as an educator.

Column 5: Put an *A* next to those that require you to administrate or direct others in a leadership position.

Column 6: Put an *A, O,* or a combination of these, next to each item, depending on whether you do it *alone* or with *others.*

Column 7: Put a *PR* next to those things that make you feel proud or good about yourself.

Column 8: Put a *V* next to those things others appreciate and value you for.

See text for a discussion of this inventory. [Adapted from Simon, S. B., Howe, L. W., & Kirschenbaum, H. *Values clarification: A handbook of strategies for teachers and students.* New York: Hart, 1972.]

Table 5-6
NURSING SKILLS INVENTORY

Clinical Skills	Management Skills	Education Skills
(List ten or more of your specialty skills. Assume basic fundamentals of nursing. If not, find a refresher.)	Leadership Planning systematically Goal setting Forecasting Policy formulation and interpretation Establishing priorities Delegation Program development Well-run meetings Supervision Hiring Firing Team building Coordinating operations Directing others Trouble shooting Evaluation Communicating effectively—listening and talking Writing—efficient, effective, and clear Organized *(Add others)*	Course design and development Course presentation clear and organized Answer questions effectively Development and explanation of evaluation process Style of presentation interesting Supervision of clinical area Positive teacher and student relationship Comfortably conduct clinical conferences Positive relationship with staff Conduct research and publish Bedside teaching clear and relevant Work cooperatively with other faculty Participates actively in co-curricular school activities Keep abreast of current trends in nursing and education Participates in faculty development Participates in professional groups contributing to professional development *(add others)*

new job because it will provide you with the opportunity to learn new skills. List three new skills you would like to learn in any of the three categories. You may desire to learn more than three skills in one category and have little or no desire to learn a skill in another category. This only points out further your leaning in one career direction.

Summary of Self-Assessments

Take time now to make a summary of what you have just learned about yourself: (1) Note your top five work values in descending order of importance. (2) List your five major work interests. Make note which ones fall into the clinical, management, or education components. (3) Make a note of the three skills that you circled in the skill assessment.

Also list the new skills you wish to learn. You might also want to note what personal or social skills you would like to be learning. Perhaps these could be learned more in one job than another. List two personal or social skills (e.g., learn to be assertive).

All of this information on choosing a career and a job path was designed to help you discover the kind of position that is best for you. Stress comes from a job–person misfit. Choosing the best job you can and keeping your career path exciting and rewarding will decrease your work stress.

Once you have the best job for yourself, you need to keep it being the best job for you. Too often nurses lapse into self-sacrificing behavior instead of setting limits by saying no. No job will remain satisfactory if you are repeatedly overloaded because you do not say no.

In summary, in analyzing your work environment for stress reduction, you need to focus on two points: what can the organization do, and what can you, as an individual nurse, do to decrease the stress? It is this person–environment fit that makes for work satisfaction.

The major conclusion to be drawn from the theoretical and research literature is that the experience of stress is caused by the person–environment misfit. Stress is a transactional process between the individual and the situation. Many studies point to the conclusion that it is not what happens out there, it is the way we perceive what happens that creates stress in our lives (Cleland, 1965; Gentry et al., 1972; Ivancevich & Matteson, 1980; Oskins, 1979).

The prevention, reduction, and treatment of stress must therefore focus on two areas. One area needing attention is the creation of an environmental atmosphere that supports health with clear work policies, adequate staffing, and responsibility in keeping with authority. Participation in decision making and recognition for a job well done are repeatedly mentioned as lacking in high-stress workplaces.

The second area of focus is the nature of the individual. Responses to any given psychosocial stimulus may vary widely from one individual to another. A study by Kobasa, Hilker, and Maddi (1979) showed that those individuals who have a sense of commitment, exercise internal control, and seek challenge or novelty will remain healthy. These traits are hard to maintain or develop in a work environment that is filled with unclear policies and limited communication.

Allen and Kraft (1981) succinctly summarize the issue of improving the quality of hospital work life for nurses:

If the nation's hospitals are going to survive their financial woes, if the nursing shortage is going to be alleviated, and hospital management problems solved, we are going to have to find ways to make hospitals highly supportive and satisfying environments for the people who work in them . . . It means primarily helping the hospital environment become one where interpersonal relationships are enjoyable, where people cooperate, where they trust each other, and where good communication is the norm. (pp. 27–28)

In the next chapter management's role in creating such an environment is explored.

6

Organizational Strategies: Improving the Organizational Climate

REVISITING THE PROBLEM

A burned-out nurse or one that is experiencing high stress levels costs the hospital in a variety of ways. The monetary cost of inefficiency is but a small portion—when this nurse is caring for a patient it is costly to a hospital in public relations and at times outright dangerous to patient safety. The high costs of turnover, absenteeism, tardiness, and continually retraining staff all add up to large problems for management. The Hospital Council of Southern California stated in a 1980 bulletin to its members that there were nurse turnover rates of 25 percent to more than 100 percent per year, recruitment costs as high as $7000 per nurse and rising, decreasing numbers of graduates and students in nursing schools, and increasing shortages in hospitals (Cunningham, 1981). Over 80 percent of American hospitals do not have adequate staffing (Aiken, 1981). Part of the reason for the 100,000 R.N. vacancies in health care facilities is that hospitals are becoming unsatisfactory places to work. Nurses call in sick, come late, or leave such environments more often now.

The short-sighted solutions of using temporary agencies and aggressive recruitment has only led to a growing unrest among existing hospital personnel. A 40 percent dropout rate, high turnover, burnout, low morale, overwork, and frustration were not problems to hospitals as long as they were able to offset attrition with a fresh supply of nurses (Kaye & Krol, 1981). Today nurses would rather switch hospitals or even careers than fight a management system that fails to deal with the causes of burnout.

Table 6-1
MAJOR WORK-RELATED STRESSORS
_____

Episodic

  Major or frequent changes in instructions, policies, or procedures.
  Major reorganization.
  Sudden significant change in the nature of the work.
  New boss or supervisor.
  Decrease in status.

Chronic

  I have unsettled conflicts with people I must work with.
  Decisions that affect me are made above, without my knowledge or
    participation.
  I lack confidence in management.
  I have too much to do and too little time to do it.
  I spend my time "fighting fires" rather than working according to a plan.
_____

Adapted from Adams, J.D. Improving stress management: An action-research-based OD intervention. In W.W. Burke (Ed.), *The cutting edges*. San Diego: University Associates, 1978.

Management's attitude toward staff members will greatly influence their level of work satisfaction. The basic concerns of management affect how the staff views management. If management is more concerned with listening to doctors' complaints than to nurses complaints, the staff knows where management's values are placed. How you are treated by management is an important factor in your work satisfaction.

Adams (1978), in his study of major sources of job-related stress, found episodic and chronic work-related stressors; they are listed in Table 6-1. Some of these are directly related to management's attitude and others are changes that need to be carefully handled to reduce the stress placed on the nurse.

There are also many studies showing the negative effects of rotating shifts (Baker, 1980; Jones, 1980; Mott, 1976; Munro, 1980; Tasto, Colligan, Skjen, & Polly, 1978; U.S. Department of Health, Education and Welfare, 1976). If nursing management does not know them, take them a copy of these articles. If nursing management does know the negative effects and is not doing anything to rectify the situation, then you have some information about management's attitude.

Management needs to change its focus to retention and career creation. Programs that demonstrate interest and sensitivity to the changing role and needs of nurses will foster better management–staff relations. The responsibility for this change lies with hospital and nursing administrations.

SIGNS OF BURNOUT IN THE ORGANIZATION

The signs of burnout in an organization fall into three categories. The first category is signs of people withdrawing from the organization. Absenteeism is a high-cost stress-linked hospital problem. The staff is habitually and deliberately not present at work. A high turnover rate is also a sign of the staff withdrawing. One study by McKenna, Oritt, and Wolff (1981) found that occupational stress is a significant predictor in the turnover decision for nurses aides and other lower level support personnel. Burke (1976) found a correlation between job satisfaction and lower levels of occupational stress.

The second category is signs of poor performance while on duty. Repeated mistakes in patient physical care (medications, irrigations) or management (prioritizing care, socioemotional, and teaching needs) spells poor performance. The patient is receiving inadequate care to promote health; the nurse feels guilty initially, but in later stages of burnout does not care.

The third category is signs of trouble in group dynamics. Lack of group cohesion, subgrouping, authoritarian leadership, etc. combine to form a stressful, low-satisfaction work climate. The lack of cohesion among faculty is a warning sign often unheeded. Johnson (1982) lists symptoms of group burnout, such as blaming the staff members, one shift blaming another, unwillingness to help, and withdrawal from other staff. Fortunately, she also offers some action steps to deal with the problem.

Withdrawal

Illness is one of the three ways of withdrawing from the organization. Obviously, when you are sick you cannot go to work. Notice if you are calling in sick more often and for illnesses you would have gone to work with 6 months ago. If so, then you are experiencing one of the withdrawal signs of organizational stress. Your stress quotient at work has exceeded your comfort zone.

As a manager, if you notice that the number and frequency of your staff calling in sick has increased, then you need to take heed of this sign. Your staff is withdrawing from work stress. The illness may also be triggered by personal stress; however, a significant number of your staff being ill should point you in the direction of examining their work units. Check your records and see if you have a significant increase in illness the past year.

Increased tardiness among your staff is also a sign of withdrawal. People are dragging themselves out of bed, but not soon enough to get to work on time. Many of these people do not see the connection between their work stress and their lateness to work. Each individual must take the responsibility of dealing with this issue, because tardiness is very disruptive to the work climate. The nurses being relieved have increased stress, as well as the manager in charge of personnel assignments. Even the nurse who is late experiences increased stress. No one comes out a winner in the tardiness game.

Millions of dollars are lost each year in health care institutions because of lateness. If a nurse is 15 minutes late twice a week and her hourly rate is $15, in 1 year she is being paid $350.00 she did not earn because she was not working. Multiply this by the number of people late and you get an idea of the high costs. Tardiness is a cost health care can no longer afford.

A high turnover rate is the third index for withdrawal, indicating a level of staff dissatisfaction. If people like their place of work they generally do not leave (other than for reasons of pregnancy, education, or relocation). Nurses leave because of poor pay, inadequate fringe benefits, or the lack of work satisfaction. The source of this dissatisfaction often is little recognition for service, limited autonomy, and policies unsupportive of nursing.

The average turnover rate for nursing personnel is 40–50 percent per year. Compare your organization to this average. If you scored better than the average, then also notice if your turnover rate has changed significantly over the past 5 years. An upward trend indicates trouble is brewing.

Poor Performance

Some nurses do not contribute to the rising turnover rate; instead, they stay and perform poorly. The cost of poor job performance cannot be measured easily. Job performance is a measure of the level of nurses' knowledge, skill, experience, and concentration. If nurses are lacking in any one of these four areas they are not performing their jobs to the best of their ability.

Nurses need to update their knowledge base continually. It is estimated that the half-life of knowledge is 5 years; for some information essential to adequate job performance it is much less. Because it is difficult to deal with this information explosion, nursing schools need to be more concerned with teaching nurses to think and problem solve, rather than only feeding them facts. The facts may change, but knowing how to gather information and think independently will help a nurse far longer than pages of facts. Knowledge of nursing theory and nursing process is just as important as knowing the normal blood pressure. Hospitals have a role in providing adequate orientation and staff development programs.

Failure on the part of health care institutions to provide adequate education leads to the stagnation of burnout. When a nurse is not performing up to par the nurse needs to assess whether more knowledge would be helpful. The organization needs to meet its responsibilities to provide a training program that supports the clinical and management skills of its personnel.

Skills, by definition, are a series of sequenced behaviors or thought processes. Skills are learned. Nurses learn mostly by watching others perform the skills. Overloaded nurses take short cuts in procedures, sometimes safely and sometimes unsafely. Students learn procedures the right way and then in the real world are forced to learn them over again. Without an adequate knowledge base new nurses may choose to take short cuts as their colleagues do in an unsafe way. Knowledge and skill training foster high standards in your organization.

When nurses are not functioning at their previous skill levels, then the chances are that some degree of burnout is present. If they fail to meet acceptable standards then they need help—either in recognizing this or in doing something to remedy the problem. Poor job performance costs everyone; the loss of self-esteem of the nurses performing poorly is a high cost.

Experience is a variable affecting job performance. New graduates are too often expected to function at a level inappropriate to their experience. Kramer and Schmalenberg (1977) called this "reality shock." If this is allowed to persist over time the stress level of these nurses will rise. Without intervention they could burn out.

Nurses need tasks appropriate to their knowledge, skill, and experience levels. A nurse who repeatedly finds herself playing in a league she is either underqualified or overqualified for will perform poorly. Educators and managers need to help nurses recognize the need for speaking up when either of these situations are occurring. If allowed to go on too long either situation creates problems in quality of care.

Finally, the level of concentration affecting job performance is the individual nurse's responsibility. Carelessness is often the result of poor concentration and this can be costly to the nurse and the patients. An intravenous line run dry, a bed rail left down, and a water pitcher left with a child who is fasting before surgery all are careless acts that hurt patients. A nurse who is overloaded has difficulty remembering the hundreds of details necessary for patient care.

A manager's decreased level of concentration shows in different ways. She forgets meetings or appointments she has set up. In counseling a staff member she cannot remember what the person said because her mind drifted off and she was not listening. She may also not be able to complete reports because of her poor concentration.

An educator's poor concentration can also show in any one of these areas. However, in the classroom the instructor needs to be attuned to the material and the students. When he or she is not, the quality of education suffers, just as the quality of care does for the practitioner.

Group Dynamics Problems

Problems in the group dynamics of the organization and the primary work group can lead to burnout. Leadership is always an issue when a group of people are together. In general, when people are tense and anxious or feel threatened in some way, they will assume either an autocratic or a laissez-faire leadership style. By either dictating or retreating, the manager-leader creates identical problems.

When managers are not available to staff or when they repeatedly take an autocratic stand, the staff feels either angry or scared; the staff's stress response is being triggered. A leader's job is to lead, and when leaders fail to lead, or dictate instead of lead, the staff feels threatened.

Remember the sign in the businessman's office, "Either lead, follow, or get out of the way." If you, as a manager, are experiencing difficulty leading, then for the sake of your staff and yourself either get training or stop being a manager. Ask yourself a career question, "Do I want to be a manager?"

Authoritarian or laissez-faire leadership also leads to a lack of group cohesion. When the staff has no leader to rally around and no leader to support the group relationship, the work unit becomes a collection of individuals. Group cohesion is a sign of an effective work group.

A faculty planning meeting is a good place to learn about the importance of group cohesion. When a group of people operate as a group they look like the Eagles going for their second touchdown pass against Dallas. They are oriented to the task and yet listening and supporting each other. A group needs to focus on its task and on its maintenance to continue to function harmoniously. A good nurse manager will recognize the need for keeping a balance. Patient care needs to get done—the manager can support this task while helping the staff to maintain positive working relationships.

Low group cohesion is a sign of organizational or work unit burnout. The group members are seen arguing, not helping each other, talking behind each other's back, and withdrawing from each other. As a manager you would know this work unit because it would be your most difficult unit to manage.

Subgrouping is a sign of lack of cohesion. Whole units (e.g., the ICU or dialysis nurses) can get designated as subgroups. Within a unit cliques form and you may hear talk of "the 3–11 or 11–7 shift," as if it were not part of the team. This and many other group dynamics problems get resolved when conflict is dealt wih openly.

All these signs lead to an overall climate of low work satisfaction for you and your staff. Think back over the last couple of years. Do you notice any change in the climate of your work unit and of your organization? What, if any, of the signs of burnout do you see in the area you are responsible for as a manager or teacher?

DETERMINING THE BURNOUT POTENTIAL OR PROBLEM

The treatment of organizational signs of burnout is best begun with a thorough examination of the organizational climate. Treatment needs to be specific and directed toward the problem area. The proper diagnosis is facilitated by the questionnaire presented in Figure 6-1.

After you have completed the questionnaire, also note the position on the dimension that would represent the majority of the nurses for which you are responsible. If you are a teacher, think about where you think your students would mark the dimensions. If you are a staff nurse, note where you believe your immediate supervisor would assess the organization.

In these seven dimensions lie the seeds of organizational burnout. The greater the difference between your ideal score and your actual score, the higher your degree of stress in that dimension. All seven dimensions contribute to either work satisfaction or the creation of burnout.

If you note a significant difference between your view of the actual situation and the other person's view you used, then note those areas. Those areas need to be addressed, otherwise poor group relations will occur, as well as the other signs of organizational burnout, such as absenteeism and poor job performance. Make note also of the discrepancies between your ideal organization and your actual organization. List the three main areas of discrepancy. Are these the same areas you noted above?

Notice the similarities and differences in the perception of the problem areas. Perhaps you can now see why your work climate is stressful. Many people find that acknowledging these differences begins to reduce the stress.

IMPROVING THE SEVEN CLIMATE DIMENSIONS

Certain policies concerning nursing practice support nurses in finding the job satisfaction possible. Management needs to educate itself to the latest findings in what facilitates an effective and satisfying work climate.

1. *Conformity:* The feeling that there are many externally imposed constraints in the organization; the degree to which members feel that there are many rules, procedures, policies, and practices to which they have to conform rather than being able to do their work as they see fit.

Conformity is not characteris- 1 2 3 4 5 6 7 8 9 10 Conformity is very characteristic
tic of the organization   _____ of the organization

2. *Responsibility:* Members of the organization are given personal responsibility to achieve their part of the organization's goals; the degree to which members feel that they can make decisions and solve problems without checking with superiors each step of the way.

No responsibility is given in 1 2 3 4 5 6 7 8 9 10 There is a great emphasis on per-
the organization   _____ sonal responsibility in the organi-
zation

3. *Standards:* The emphasis the organization places on quality performance and outstanding production, including the degree to which the member feels the organization is setting challenging goals for itself and communicating these goal commitments to members.

Standards are very low or 1 2 3 4 5 6 7 8 9 10 High, challenging standards are
nonexistent in the organiza- _____ set in the organization
tion

4. *Rewards:* The degree to which members feel that they are being recognized and rewarded for good work, rather than being ignored, criticized, or punished when something goes wrong.

Members are ignored, pun- 1 2 3 4 5 6 7 8 9 10 Members are recognized and re-
ished or criticized   _____ warded positively

5. *Organizational clarity:* The feeling among members that things are well organized and goals are clearly defined rather than being disorderly, confused, or chaotic.

The organization is disorderly, 1 2 3 4 5 6 7 8 9 10 The organization is well organized
confused, and chaotic   _____ with clearly defined goals

6. *Warmth and support:* The feeling that friendliness is a valued norm in the organization; that members trust one another and offer support to one another. The feeling that good relationships prevail in the work environment.

There is no warmth and sup- 1 2 3 4 5 6 7 8 9 10 Warmth and support are very char-
port in the organization   _____ acteristic of the organization

7. *Leadership:* The willingness of organization members to accept leadership and direction from qualified others. As needs for leadership arise members feel free to take leadership roles and are rewarded for successful leadership. Leadership is based on expertise. The organization is not dominated by, or dependent on, one or two individuals.

Leadership is not rewarded: 1 2 3 4 5 6 7 8 9 10 Members accept and reward lead-
members are dominated or de- _____ ership based on expertise
pendent and resist leadership
attempts

FIGURE 6-1. Organizational climate questionnaire. For each of the seven organizational climate dimensions described, place an "A" below the number that indicates your assessment of the organization's current position on that dimension and an "I" below the number that indicates your choice of where the organization ideally should be on this dimension. [Reprinted from Kolb, D. A., Rubin, I. M., & McIntyre, J. M. *Organizational psychology: An experimental approach* (3rd ed.). © 1979, pp. 193–194. With permission of Prentice-Hall, Englewood Cliffs, N.J.]

Conformity

If a high degree of conformity is demanded, nurses often experience a lack of mental challenge. Obviously, policies and procedures are necessary, otherwise a decision would have to be made over and over again. Workers who feel that their suggestions are influential in shaping policies (Daley, 1979) and that they play a meaningful part in the administrative decisions affecting their work (Pines & Kafry, 1978) are more satisfied with their work climate. Rules are short cuts for thinking; they are not meant to override or discourage flexible thinking.

Policies need to be supportive of a high degree of autonomy in nursing practice (Mundinger, 1980). Policies that support nonnursing duties or authoritarian decision making do not lead to a feeling of being treated as an intelligent, contributing member of the organization. Autonomy and independence in nursing practice are key issues in preventing burnout. It is important to allow nurses to do their work as they see fit according to the standards of nursing practice. In some hospitals the standards imposed by hospital rules and policies severely limit the nurse in performing at her highest skill level.

Conformity problems are treated by decentralizing decision making. If you, as a manager, see your staff as capable and competent to make decisions autonomously, then you do not need to impose burdensome restraints on their autonomy. If management does not see staff as capable, then the staff need support in learning this skill.

A common cry I hear from frustrated nurses is that management makes the decisions but is not close enough to the issues to have the kind of information needed for effective decisions. Participative decision making offers the staff or the students an opportunity to take a role in the decisions affecting them. Policies and procedures supportive of quality nursing care need to be clear; when they are not supportive, but inhibiting, then they need to be changed.

Emphasis on unit-based leadership allows for more autonomy in nursing practice. Having clinical specialists available to support the staff's clinical decision making is likely to increase job satisfaction. Primary nursing reduces the level of decision making to the most appropriate level for the patient (Zander, 1980). Conformity to certain restraints is necessary; however, autonomy of practice is equally necessary. A stress prevention system could include a clinical career ladder with increasing levels of autonomy to reward the nurse for increasing her clinical skill level.

Responsibility

Responsibility is sometimes also called accountability. The most important aspect of being responsible or accountable is that with it must come the authority to carry out the responsibility. Frustration, resentment, and signs of burnout will follow if a nurse is repeatedly put in a responsible position and not given the tools of authority and resources to carry out the responsibility. If managers require staff to check repeatedly with them on decisions, then they are creating a dependent staff and probably a frustrated one.

Dr. Linda Aiken, in her presidential address at the 1980 meeting of the American Academy of Nursing, spoke about the issue of responsibility without authority. Under the present hospital system, nurses get 24-hour responsibility for patient care, but little authority. She listed six reasons this system is no longer satisfactory for nurses (Aiken, 1981):

- Increased demand on nurses for technological and clinical expertise
- Increased complexity of patient needs
- Growth of subspecialty medicine, which contributes to the fragmentation of care
- Reduced work weeks for American workers, including physicians
- Increased career aspirations of women
- Little recognition of the importance of nurses' role in the new level of clinical decision making.

These factors alone could provide justification for giving nurses the authority for the responsibility they have had for years.

The Ivancevich and Matteson (1980) survey pointed to responsibility as an important job stressor. The five most stressful areas were responsibility for people, time pressures, role conflict, relationships with other nurses, and relationships with supervisors; four of the five deal directly with relationship and responsibility issues.

The success stories at the National Commission on Nursing meeting ("Initial report," 1981) clearly pointed to having nurses more involved in decisions that affect them directly. Nurse participation on all hospital and medical staff committees and in the selection of the medical staff is an example of nurses getting some authority over issues for which they may be responsible.

Anderson and Basteyns (1981) studied 182 full-time ICU nurses and found that the major ICU stressors were all externally controlled. The stressors were staffing problems, the heavy work load, and communication difficulties with physicians. It has long been recommended that the nurse–patient ratio in critical care units be 1:2. A 4–40 work pattern was also suggested for staffing problems and to allow time for recovery time. In this system a person works four 10-hour days and then has off three days in succession. These problems need to be addressed otherwise nurses will continue to feel helpless and therefore increasingly stressed in the presence of such external factors.

Management needs to consider the significant stress it places on an individual who is responsible for running an efficient and effective work unit but does not have the authority to do so. The authority determining who works on that unit (hiring and firing), dealing with repeated personal problems with an employee (disciplining), or determining the type and amount of equipment needed for patient care (budget) is key in preventing job stress. Management needs to decide how decentralized it wants the organization to be. To keep decision making at its lowest level, the responsibility of running a nurses' unit should be placed with the people who know that work unit best—the staff. What the various levels of the nursing hierarchy have the responsibility to decide depends on the leadership style of the management.

Standards

Clearly defined measurements of quality performance carried out by the staff lead to excellent patient care. When quality performance is expected and justly rewarded by management, the staff feels challenged by the goals. Participating in the formulation of these standards would involve staff in the decision-making process on a meaningful level. Involving staff in decisions helps prevent rebellion and the feeling of being "left out" or "not consulted" (Veninga, 1982). Clinical career ladders help reinforce the notion of quality nursing standards. A collaborative practice committee composed of nurses and physicians is a symbol of the goal of quality patient care. Opportunities for research and publication on clinical nursing care help support the norm of quality care.

When nurses look to their clinical superior for a role model and find standards of nursing practice that do not support quality patient care, then they feel the standards of their organization are in need of change. Nursing teachers need to remember they, too, are role models for quality nursing graduates. If you are not clear about what your nursing standards are, then you have some homework to do.

Working according to your nursing care standards is like living according to your value system. Both help reduce stress by providing boundaries for your comfort zone. Not living according to your nursing standards or working in an organization with low standards creates the stress of internal conflict.

Many standards of health care are changing. One such change is exemplified by the fact that 400 hospitals have developed health promotion and prevention programs. Their wellness programs are the new standards promoted by these hospitals. Unfortunately, nurses have gotten little credit for the importance of their role in creating the wellness movement. Nursing standards of patient education finally paid off with the consumer demanding information and health care skills.

Rewards

Of all the dimensions, reward surfaces as a problem with a resounding roar in most organizations. Business and industry are way ahead of health care in this dimension. Their workers are not expected to rely on the internal altruistic reward that nurses are expected to depend upon. Management could probably afford to be more generous with the recognition of staff; the same goes for most teachers, actually for most people. If replenishing recognition does not come from the top, then down the ladder there are probably even larger deficiencies in recognition.

Recognition comes in two forms: (1) salary and benefits, and (2) verbal–nonverbal recognition. Salaries have certainly increased, and so have benefit packages. Several authors (Daley, 1979; Pines & Kafry, 1978; Ramprasad, 1973) have noted low salaries as a source of work stress. Unfortunately, the verbal–nonverbal recognition has not increased proportionately. This lack of recognition has been cited by a number of authors (Daley, 1979; Emener, 1979; Pines & Kafry, 1978; Ramprasad, 1973; Veninga, 1979).

Feeling appreciated by those you work for and with makes it inviting to come to work. When work is a place to get recognized and rewarded you do not want to take days off or leave your workplace. When people leave work dissatisfied they are usually "stroke" deprived. Verbal thank yous and acknowledgments of a job well done, along with nonverbal smiles of recognition, do a lot to give the staff a sense of achievement. Written letters and notes of positive performance, along with recognition in the organizational newsletter, can motivate staff to higher and higher levels of quality care. Recognition of work employment, anniversary, and birthdates gives the staff conditional and unconditional recognition. This recognition also helps create an atmosphere of warmth and support.

Organizational Clarity

The members of an organization need to be clearly aware of the goals, policies, and procedures of the organization. All levels of management need to be responsible for clearly communicating these to nurses for whom they are responsible. Without organizational clarity role conflict and role ambiguity occur. Role conflict and role ambiguity are seen as a source of work stress by many authors (Daley, 1979; Ivancevich & Matteson, 1980; Munro, 1980; Veninga, 1979).

Role conflict is best treated by clarifying what expectations different people have of you. If you try to live up to conflicting expectations stress problems are sure to ensue.

Role ambiguity is best treated with a clear job description and clarification of this description with your immediate superior. Clarification is also important with the nurses for whom you are responsible. A lot of anger and resentment could be avoided if people stopped assuming and instead clarified their roles. Role ambiguity in our age of specialization is a real problem; nursing roles need continuous clarification.

Rules reduce uncertainty and prevent the chaos of "everybody doing their own thing." Management needs to determine and enforce rules, and yet also be open to redefining them when appropriate. Rules, policy, and procedures are designed to promote organizational clarity, not produce stress because they are inflexible and antiquated.

Warmth and Support

Co-workers need to be able to trust and support one another. According to Erickson (1968), the development of trust is basic to individual development and without it all other developmental stages lie on shaky ground. A trusting work environment provides the staff with a basis for good working relationships. If you cannot trust the nurse you work with and feel you cannot count on him or her for help, then your workday will contain significant anxiety.

The group dynamics of subgrouping and scapegoating need to be treated to allow an atmosphere of trust to develop. A staff will break into subgroups or project the cause of the problem onto an individual when open discussion of differences is not allowed. If I am able to voice disagreement with you then I will not have to tell it to someone else. A warm, supportive work environment is the result of keeping communication channels open for positive and negative feedback. Upper levels of nursing set the tone; you are the role models for warmth and support. To prevent the overload of the stress of daily work activities, staff members need to talk about their feelings openly and receive the kind of emotional replenishment they need. As a faculty member, when was the last time you shared your feelings on an issue?

Support groups can do much to reduce work stress. They provide a protective buffer against work pressure. One of the most crucial elements in staff morale is whether there are good working relationships among colleagues (Pines & Kafry, 1978). Supportive work groups, where responsibilities are shared, are experienced by professionals as less personally stressful. Support from others enriches the resources available on the job.

Several studies have offered specific suggestions for ICUs to decrease

Table 6-2
MEASURES TO INCREASE SUPPORT IN THE ICU

Schools of nursing need to incorporate both theoretical and clinical ICU experience into the curriculum.

Inservice programs need to be offered for ICU staff.

Death, grief, and mourning process education programs plus discussion sessions to ventilate feelings need to be instituted (Huckabay & Jagla, 1979, p. 26).

Regular forums need to be held for discussion of issues involving strong feelings, such as who should be resuscitated.

Forums should be held where experienced and advanced knowledge could be shared with all personnel.

Charge, teaching, and orienting duties need to be designed to minimize interstaff competition.

Selection of new nurses and new head nurses should be shared by the staff (Cassem & Hackett, 1975, p. 258).

Nurses should receive 6 weeks of comprehensive specialty training prior to beginning work on a unit (pathophysiologic parameters, psychological aspects of critical care, need for cooperative team, explanation of unit policies, and instruction about equipment and procedures).

There should be a full-time physician director of the CCU with whom the head nurse can actively facilitate the resolution of conflicts between nurses and physicians.

Involve families in care of the patients.

Reinforce a sense of accomplishment in patient care by inquiring about patient's status after they leave the unit (Gardner et al., 1980, pp. 104–105).

Insist upon training in the field of critical care for nursing supervisors who are responsible for ICU areas.

Include stress management and humanistic approaches in training for nursing personnel.

Place seasoned, experienced nurses on the staff of critical care units.

Develop methods to measure attrition rates, absenteeism, request for transfer, and intrastaff conflicts which may be indicators of the occupational stress levels (Hoffman, 1981).

---

stress and increase support; they are listed in Table 6-2. Many of these suggestions for an ICU staff would be equally applicable to other hospital units.

Leadership

Since the first classic studies in the 1930s, leadership has become a much researched subject that is still not well understood. The early study by Lewin, Lippitt, and White (1939) revealed dramatic differences in behavioral and emotional aspects of group process as a consequence of autocratic, democratic, or laissez-faire styles of leadership. Since that time two major types of leadership behaviors have been studied, variously labeled as autocratic versus democratic (Shaw, 1955), task oriented versus human relations oriented (Katz & Kahn, 1952), and distant, controlling, managing versus psychologically close, permissive (Fiedler, 1967). Experimental findings have been inconsistent; often no statistically significant difference is observed.

Hershey and Blanchard (1977) have a slightly different focus and state that the style of leadership needs to be dependent upon the situation. The kinds of behavior associated with each style demonstrate the flexibility needed for effective leadership. Individuals choosing the first style have a high need for structure. They tend to make the decisions and then tell subordinates what to do. Individuals with the second style take a collaborative or participative approach. With a greater orientation toward people, they tend to typify the "let's do it together" attitude. A consultative approach is a third style. People with this style give other people the responsibility and then act as a resource for them. The fourth style, in its extreme, looks like laissez-faire leadership. These leaders provides little structure for tasks and little socioemotional support for the people. They delegate the work and "let people do what they want." You can see how each of these four behavior styles can be effective or ineffective in different situations. Flexible leaders have the potential to be effective in a number of situations (Drucker, 1967; Hart, 1980).

Your style needs to be adaptable. Leadership flexibility is necessary in complex managerial jobs involving rapid environmental change and many interconnecting jobs. Nursing is such a job. To obtain a more detailed analysis of this way of looking at leadership and also to gain information on how to increase your flexibility, read *Management of Organizational Behavior: Utilizing Human Resources* by Hershey and Blanchard (1977). They offer a nurse manager the concise information necessary to understand the interaction of people, motivation, and leadership (Stevens, 1980).

Leadership problems need to be addressed in two domains. First, qualified leaders need to be developed and then allowed to exert their due influence. Second, leaders need to be acknowledged and rewarded for their managing skills. Leadership is both a cause and an effect of the other seven dimensions.

Management training fosters leadership qualities and skills. The skills of an effective leader need to be taught on all levels, beginning at the top and working down to staff nurse levels. This training needs to be continuous and appropriate for the various hierarchy levels. It should include recognizing stress signs in the staff and the organization. In order to prevent and reduce the stress of both the manager and the staff nurse or student, they need to develop certain skills.

Table 6-3
THE SUCCESSFUL LEADER

Gives clear work instructions; communicates well in general; keeps others informed

Praises others when they deserve it; understands the importance of recognition; looks for opportunities to build the esteem of others

Is willing to take time to listen to others; is sensitive to the powerful effect of good leadership listening both for building a cooperative relationship and avoiding tension and grievances

Is cool and calm most of the time; maintains emotional control in almost any situation; can be counted on to behave maturely and appropriately

Has confidence and self-assurance

Has appropriate technical knowledge of the work being supervised; uses this knowledge to coach, teach, and evaluate rather than for getting involved in the "doing" of the work

Understands the group's problems; demonstrates this by careful and attentive listening and by honestly trying to project into their situation

Gains the group's respect; this is accomplished through personal honesty with the group, avoidance of trying to appear more knowledgeable than is true, and having no fear of saying "I don't know" or "I made a mistake"

Is fair to everyone; this is demonstrated through patterns of work assignments, consistent enforcement of rules, policies, and procedures, and avoidance of favoritism

Demands good work from everyone; maintains consistent standards of performance; will not expect the work group to "take up the slack" for a "lazy" worker; enforces work discipline

Gains the people's trust; this is demonstrated by the leader's willingness to represent the group to "higher management," regardless of agreement or disagreement with them, the leader "carries their message"

Goes to bat for the group; will work for the best and fair interests of the work group; will not shrink from approaching higher management when necessary; has loyalties to both higher management and the work group

"Is not stuck up"; maintains a relationship of friendliness while remembering he or she is not "one of the guys"—this is a difficult distinction to make

"Is easy to talk to"; demonstrates a desire to understand without shutting off feedback through scolding, judging, moralizing, or belittling

---

Adapted from Jennings, E. *An anatomy of Leadership: Princes, heroes, and supermen.* New York: McGraw-Hill, 1972.

The leadership skills listed in Table 6-3 are based on the 14 traits and skills that have been shown to be characteristic of successful leaders. These items were identified through extensive research done by Dr. Eugene E. Jennings of Michigan State University. As you read the list, note those traits or skills that you feel you possess.

Note your assets as well as your liabilities. Perhaps you could reduce considerable stress by developing some of these qualities in yourself. Whatever your nursing function, some level of leadership is necessary. By fostering leadership skills in yourself and others you will ultimately improve the quality of patient care and increase the level of professionalism in nursing.

SUGGESTIONS OF THE NATIONAL COMMISSION ON NURSING

The National Commission on Nursing, which was established in Fall of 1980, is sponsored by the American Hospital Association, Hospital Research and Education Trust, and American Hospital Supply Corporation. The commission is charged with the task of exploring the causes and effects of and potential solutions to the current nursing-related problems. At hearings in six cities individual nurses spoke of their frustrations and the professional changes they wanted. One of the issues addressed by the commission's 24 preliminary recommendations was lack of collaboration ("Initial Report," 1981). Commission Chairman H. Robert Cathcart, president of Pennsylvania Hospital, said that the commission found that while nurses are accountable for nursing care, they lack necessary decision-making authority. The recommendations call for nurses to be part of the clinical decision process in a collaborative relationship with physicians.

In a March 1982 meeting, representatives of 32 hospitals considered to have nursing success stories got together to share their ideas. Four-member teams—nurse administrator, physician, chief executive officer, and trustee—were present from each hospital. The purpose of that meeting was to seek information about organizational structures and management techniques that promote quality care, enhance relationships among the groups represented, and make nursing careers more satisfying.

Representatives of seven hospitals made presentations describing approaches they had found to be effective in improving the environment for nursing care. Responses of a survey, which had been sent to all participants previously, were also a source for discussion; 72 percent of the respondents reported a decrease in nursing turnover.

This record showed that they could adapt and adjust to changes. It was evident to all that the problems related to nursing were part of the problems of the broader health care system. The description of these hospitals unfortunately will sound Utopian to many nurses.

Joyce Clifford, Vice President for Nursing at Beth Israel Hospital in Boston cited changes that strongly affected the direction of nursing in her hospital over an 8-year period (McCarty, 1982):

Table 6-4
ASSESSING ORGANIZATIONAL POLICIES

Collaborative practice committees composed of nurses and physicians.
Clinical and administrative career ladders for nurses.
Clinical specialists to support staff nurse decision making.
Emphasis on team building, problem solving, and conflict resolution techniques.
Flexible and innovative scheduling.
Patient acuity-based staffing.
Internship program for new nurses.
Management seminars for all levels of nurses.
Increased percentage of RNs on staff.
Nurse participation on all hospital and medical staff committees.
Improved salary and benefits with incentives for clinical leadership.
Nursing representation on hospital committees proportionate to the number of
    employees.
Participation of the work group involved in the interviewing and selecting of head
    nurses and other nurse managers.
Participation of nurses in the selection of medical staff.

Reprinted from McCarty, P. Hospitals share success stories. *The American Nurse,* 1981, *14*
(5), pp. 1, 7, 17. With permission.

- Primary nursing
- Unit-based leadership and unit-based activities
- Position of head nurse as full manager of her unit
- Recognition throughout the hospital of primary role of nursing in pa-
  tient care and decision making
- Opportunity for nurses to advance their professionalism through publi-
  cation, research, and committee activity.

This upgraded view of nursing was a common practice among participants. Many nursing administrators had direct access to the board of
trustees.

   Many hospitals had decreased the layers of the organizational structure between the top administrator and the head nurses. At several hospitals, only a layer of assistants, responsible for a clinical area or responsible for a management function, existed between the head nurses and the
nursing administrator.

   Fourteen other changes that supported nursing were cited by conference participants. They are listed in Table 6-4; note those that are presently being developed or are implemented in your organization.

   The participants were urged by representatives of the smaller hospitals to keep the needs of small, rural hospitals in mind. Over 50 percent

of the hospitals belonging to the American Hospital Association have less than 100 beds.

Nurse administrators compiled a list of 52 concerns involved in improving the environment for nursing practice. Condensed, they are represented by five major concerns (McCarty, 1982, pp. 7, 14):

- Reimbursement constraints that limit the quality care available to patients;
- Lack of cohesiveness in the profession resulting in inability to move forward;
- Conflicts between the new societal values held by many recent graduates and the traditional expectations of hospitals;
- Inadequacies in the educational system; and
- Lack of understanding among health professions, resulting in turf battles.

Dr. M. Aydelotte, former executive director of the ANA, made several interesting points in her address to the commission (Initial report and preliminary recommendations of the National Commission on Nursing, 1981). She spoke of the change in peoples' orientation to work. People today are seeking meaning in their work. They desire recognition and a challenge in what they do. They want involvement, more participation, and autonomy in work. Today's workers do not readily accept authority and a passive role. Relationships have become strained. She emphasized the importance of resolving relationships among professionals.

The commission members expressed their hope that this meeting would be a turning point. Nursing is certainly a pivotal point in the changing health care system. The conference participants—three-fourths of them from outside the profession of nursing—successfully addressed the issues that directly and indirectly affect the stress levels of nurses.

Robert Feldman, a trustee of Mount Sinai Medical Center, Miami Beach, Florida, suggested that all trustees read the *Summary of Public Hearings* and the *Initial Report and Preliminary Recommendations of the National Commission on Nursing* (1981). I make a similar suggestion to you.*

The commission points out that nursing is an integral part of the dynamic and complex health care system in the United States. The commission will focus on creating four outcomes: (1) retention of nurses in practice, (2) job satisfaction, (3) maintaining and increasing the competence of nurses in practice, and (4) maintaining and improving the quality of nursing care. All four would be facilitated with a nurse having a comfortable level of stress under which to function.

---

*Order through the American Hospital Association, 840 North Lake Shore Drive, Chicago, IL 60611.

HIGH-RISK PROFILE FOR BURNOUT IN
MANAGERS

Managers, please take note of the following results from a 3-year British Study conducted on 500 male managers. Melhuish and Cooper have developed a high-risk profile emphasizing six sets of factors:

1. High need to succeed. Probably a workaholic, preoccupied with meeting deadlines.
2. Conflict between personal and company values. Seems to feel that the company continually asks him to choose between company and family.
3. Sees his company as dominated by politics and competition.
4. Superiors and peers put heavy demands on his time and talents.
5. Feels high job insecurity.
6. A final cluster of equally influential factors—intelligence, suspiciousness, apprehensiveness, a serious nature, and general tension—also helps to characterize the high-stress illness group. ("Study Tracking Stress Response," 1981, p. 87)

If any of these factors belong to you, take heed and begin a program to reduce your high risk. To correct some of these factors the environment needs alteration, and for other factors the manager's basic personality needs to change. Attention to these factors reduces your chance of burnout. As an educator or practitioner you may also notice these characteristics as part of your profile.

Responsibility for others can be very stressful without the necessary skills. Developing the skills discussed in the next section will help you reduce your risk of burnout.

MANAGEMENT SKILLS NEEDED TO PREVENT
BURNOUT

All aspects of nursing require some degree of the management skills of planning, organizing, directing, and controlling. Reducing, treating, and preventing your work stress depends on your developing these skills. The reduction of stress often occurs when the individual goes from a state of uncertainty to certainty. Knowing what is expected of you in a role as a manager will alert you to the problems you need to address and the skills you need to learn. As a health care coordinator you perform the acts of a manager—planning, organizing, directing, and controlling.

Most of the material in this section on the tasks of a manager is taken from Arndt and Huckabay (1980). These authors clearly describe the process of managing; each dimension is related to stress.

Planning

Health care institutions are complex because they involve many interdependencies. For the flexibility necessary for a continuously changing environment, a structure low in formality is best. Planning at levels where individuals see the problems with the most clarity is prevented with a very formal structure. Planning requires a number of skills and is needed on all hierarchical levels for an organization to function effectively.

The process of planning starts with the collection and interpretation of the facts; subsequently an action-oriented plan is developed based on these facts. Because your own biasing experiences and the effects of stress distort your perceptions, it is difficult to keep this process objective. However, forecasting the future and deciding on which steps to take requires as much objectivity as you can muster. Next you need to set up a plan to carry out your proposed action and a monitoring system to check on the plan's effectiveness.

The planning process, according to Arndt and Huckabay (1980), unfolds in seven interdependent phases. These phases may occur together, and all are considered in a systems approach to planning.

In order to develop an inclusive, flexible plan, the manager needs to be thinking in long-range terms. Long-range thinking helps the manager in two ways: (1) By seeing the organization as a whole, rather than just parts, the manager is likely to plan strategies, rather than just try to correct idividual, immediate problems. (2) It is necessary to define performance measures for the system to evaluate the workability of the strategies.

Managers need to question whether they are assessing *their* present state of affairs or their organization's present state. Too often managers allow themselves to decrease their stress level through immediate gratification of their needs, rather than by developing long-term stress reducers. When you know the state of yourself and your organization, only then can you answer the question, "What are my goals?" The first stage, therefore, is the assessment of the organization in its present state.

The formulation of organizational and individual goals is the second stage. Subsequent steps are prioritized for each goal. For instance, reflect for a moment on the priority of having a healthy life—a satisfying job. Developing a stress course for the freshman students (organizational goal) would teach you the guidelines of a healthy life (personal goal) and might even make your job more satisfying. Time deadlines for completion are determined for each goal and each step.

In the third stage you assess your larger organizational capabilities and potentialities. Your individual planning can be accurate only if you have some idea of your organizational goals and assets. As a head nurse, you may need to look at the nursing service system, whereas as a teacher you would be assessing the college of nursing or even the medical science department. As the picture comes into focus, the resources, strengths, weaknesses, opportunities, and constraints present themselves.

Both the actual physical environment and the social environment are assessed. The communication patterns of the department staff, as well as the interrelationship with other departments are examined. Too often, assessment of the people issues (conflict, leadership) is overlooked or not seen as important. Conflictual interpersonal relationships increase work stress and are therefore very important in this assessment process.

Forecasting begins at this stage. The manager develops a plan based on a projected realistic picture of the system's strengths and weaknesses. A plan based on forecasts consisting only of ideals is doomed to failure. For example, a 350-bed metropolitan hospital developed and designed a wellness program based on two ideals: that people will take responsibility for their health given the opportunity to engage in good nutrition, physical fitness, and stress management programs; and that once they have taken that opportunity, they will continue to do so when you remove the incentives of time off, money, and peer pressure. Need I say that management failed to forecast accurately the outcome of the program. Good forecasting would consider the nursing shortage or the need for a nursing education program to be holistic in its approach.

The fourth stage is beginning to determine how the goals will be reached. The manager may be considering the implementation of primary care nursing or a video patient education program. Factors are weighed, such as the cost–effectiveness ratio, the acceptability to staff or patients, and the urgency of the goal or objective. Plans become specific as alternatives are weeded out. The necessary procedures to implement action are begun. This is one of the high-stress times in an organization because individuals are in a state of anticipation. Managers could significantly reduce this stress by having staff involved and informed; information reduces the fear of the unknown.

Even though this stage is still not an action-taking stage, it involves a great deal of collaborative effort with staff. Too often, inadequately planned courses or programs fall through and this creates tension and disappointment for students and staff.

In stage five priorities are established. They depend upon the organization's obligation, the impact of the service being planned, and the readiness of the community. For example, is the community ready for a nurse practitioner master's program, can the university afford the program, and what will the impact be on physician–nurse relationships?

The sequence of the program activities needs to be considered carefully. For example, consider the planning and the organizing of a wellness curriculum. The lead time involves the education of faculty and the public relations aspect of the program. The initial trial period covers the beginning of implementation of the program; it is followed by a peak load adjustment. As mentioned previously, this adjustment period is a most difficult time. The program may end up getting scrapped completely if the necessary evaluation procedures were not established. (Remember the last diet that got dropped rather than evaluated, or the last management course?)

Implementation is the sixth stage. For example, a commitment is made to develop a nursing wellness program and the resources are allocated. Here, the educator acts as the stage director, actively partaking or delegating. A manager will encounter many resistances to and conflicts with the change; they are to be expected. The manager needs to consider this in choosing implementation procedures. Staff involvement in your planning is guaranteed to reduce resistance. As a manager, remember a resistant staff raises your stress level.

The seventh stage involves the evaluation and surveillance of the plan. The evaluation system instituted needs to provide feedback on the outcomes measured against the objectives. The evaluation plan needs to have periodic progress checks. These checks provide the feedback that would be lost in final evaluation.

Perfectionists often have trouble with this stage because the mistakes show and this raises their stress level. Seeing mistakes as feedback rather than judgments has reduced many a perfectionist's blood pressure. Evaluation seen as grades rather than as an assessment process is likely to raise the stress level of all concerned.

The major characteristics of a good plan are summarized in eight dimensions by Arndt and Huckabay (1980). Answer the questionnaire presented in Table 6-5 to assess your planning skill at present. Think of a recent time your were required to make a major plan, professionally or personally. It needs to have been significant enough so that you can assess yourself in all the important dimensions. Respond with either a "yes" or a "no."

How many questions did you answer "yes"? How many "no"? Consider the areas in which you answered "no." You need to improve your planning skills in these areas. The sources of stress in planning result from the constantly changing external environment. The requirements for the role of a nurse manager are also changing, and these changes create the stress of role conflict. Assessing a system in which you work is a difficult

Table 6-5
EXAMINING YOUR PLANNING

1. Was the plan based on clearly defined objectives that were as clear to you as they were to those who were concerned with the implementation and operation of the plan?
2. Was the plan clear and simple, not ambiguous?
3. Did the plan provide for stability and flexibility? Could people trust the stability of your plan, yet see that the plan was capable of adaptation?
4. Was the plan economical and realistic in terms of the resources needed? Did you exercise the principle of economy in the use of funds, equipment, supplies, personnel, energy, etc.?
5. Were the means to accomplish the plan and evaluation standards clear? Was the plan operationally defined and was it evaluated against standards?
6. Did the plan anticipate the future and consider the input from forecasts of the future? Did you consider economic and political variables, patient needs, and the changing social environment?
7. Was the plan purposeful, rational, and justifiable in terms of objectives?
8. Did the plan allow for the unique sociopolitical environment of the organization? Was your plan politically and socially wise?

Adapted from Arndt, C., & Huckabay, L. *Nursing administration: Theory for practice with a systems approach.* St. Louis: Mosby, 1980.

task to do objectively, yet effort needs to be directed toward reducing some of the stress of uncertainty.

Planning is a skill that requires assessing and diagnosing the system and developing goals and action steps for the present and future. Performing this function without adequate information and skill is stressful for any nurse.

Organizing

Organizing skill is needed to manage an organization or to manage yourself. Creating a structure that allows for maximum productivity, job satisfaction, or student learning involves organizing. Having determined your objectives, you then group activities, delineate authority and responsibility, and establish working relationships to accomplish the goal.

Coordination is another word for organization. A patient care coordinator is a nurse who organizes the nursing unit so that quality patient care ensues and the staff enjoys its work. Many interedepartmental misunderstandings could be avoided if more importance were given to coordination.

ARE YOU WORKING IN A SUCCESSFUL
ORGANIZATION?

Studies have shown that there are six essential components of a successful organization. (Arndt & Huckabay, 1980, p. 74):

- Strong resourceful leadership
- Clearly defined responsibilities
- Carefully selected, trained, and placed working force
- Standardized methods
- Adequate cost effectiveness and records
- Cooperation.

How many are part of your organization? They are *all* fundamental for effective organizing.

Stieglitz (1971) lists four elements of organizing: objectives; activities or groups of activities; authority; and relationships. The principles arising from these elements are not meant as dogma, rather they are meant as guides.

Objectives need to be consistent and clear on all levels. They should be written so that they can be referred to as necessary. Each nursing unit or nursing curriculum must be guided in a common direction, otherwise the stress of confusion will arise. If your professional as well as personal goals are consistent you will reduce stress. For instance, effective managing and playing favorites is inconsistent, as is maintaining good health and smoking. With clear and direct objectives, any deviation will be a significant deviation, not just a slight exception that can be overlooked. Clear guidelines reduce the stress of role conflict and of role ambiguity.

There are many ways to design and group activities in organizing. Whatever the organization decides is the way to group activities will define to some degree what you will do or not do in your nursing practice. When nursing activities are grouped according to a functional approach, the interdependency aspects need to be attended to. If primary nursing is the approach, the head nurse would group patients differently.

Another approach to grouping activities is exemplified by the increasing trend toward decentralized nursing departments. Decentralization involves delegating authority and responsibility for decisions as close to the scene of action as possible. Having the authority to carry out decisions decreases the stress involved in responsibility. Decentralization frees up the individual manager to concentrate on a broader scope for his or her nursing practice.

Arndt and Huckabay (1980) list three criteria that need to be considered in delegating decision making: competence of the individual, information available, and the scope of the impact of the decision. Having the freedom to delegate without a competent individual to delegate to raises, rather than lowers, stress. Furthermore, sometimes a manager is unable to act because the administration is withholding information. Decentralization in practice is a matter of the degree of decision making allowed.

Nurses who are poor in delegating responsibility will feel stressed when confronted with the prospect of increased decentralization. However, with training in the appropriate skills, nurses can greatly reduce the stress of overload. In the long run, stress levels will be reduced with decentralization because nurses will experience more control over their work environment; the stress of uncertainty will be decreased. Delegation is an important skill and will be addressed again in the next section.

The third element of organizational planning is the delineation of authority. We experience authority through demonstrating our leadership. In your position as an authority someone will be superior and someone will be subordinate to you. Sometimes your authority is based on your position and if you leave the position you loose the authority. Your authority is also based upon your expertise, an important fact that nurses forget.

In your position as an authority you have the right to delegate or to act on certain decisions. Even though you may not be involved with the actual policy-making decision, you may need to operate on and enforce the decision. Stress is reduced when your values concerning authority agree with your organization.

When an organization is organized clearly and definitely, everyone knows their line of staff relationships. Knowing who is responsible for what reduces role ambiguity. A *line authority* is the person held accountable for the desired result. The staff person is responsible to supply the information that will enable this accountable nurse to make the best decision. If the lines of authority are not clear, anxiety is created due to role conflict or role ambiguity.

Another way of looking at the organizing of authority relations is by viewing "line" and "lateral" as the types of authority. In your line relationships you are directly and immediately responsible to your line authority, whereas with your lateral health care personnel you are involved in no direct authority. The dietician and the pharmacist, for example, are not your line authorities. Take time to write down the hierarchy of your organization. Start with your director of nursing and work down to your position. Connect all the line relationships with a solid line and all the lateral relationships with dotted lines. If you find any authority relationships that are not clear to you, find out who is responsible to whom.

Several factors determine each person's working relationships with others. The formal structure, designated by the organizational chart, is one of the organizational tools to define relationships. The informal structure and the communication process are less tangible ways of defining working relationships. The informal communication channels, such as the "hospital grapevine," do a lot to define relationships. Zander (1977) cites a 1962 study showing that poor communication within a hospital damages collaboration among staff members and makes the organization less efficient.

If you work in a large system it is likely that you are unfamiliar with the whole organizational pattern. It is often difficult for the staff to feel the effectiveness of their contribution in a large system. When managers provide recognition by involving staff on hospital committees, they begin to understand and impact the organization as a whole. This involvement helps them see how changes occur in the organization, and serves to reduce alienation.

The informal structure represents the social relationships, the power figures, and the social norms of the organization. This informal system also defines "the person to see" and "the way to get things done here." When these two systems differ significantly the organization is usually highly stressful.

Allen and Kraft (1981) point out the importance of knowing the social norms present in a work environment; these norms are "the accepted, expected, and supported ways of behaving" (p. 20). They state, "These norms—most often unwritten and largely unrecognized—are powerful determinants of what happens" (p. 20). Norms form the standard operating procedures for the informal structure.

How do you know your norms, both the positive and the negative ones? Just listen and watch and you can hear and see the norms in action. For example, hearing nurses repeatedly talk about nurses in other departments behind their backs indicates that backbiting is a communication norm. Seeing nurses giving each other positive recognition and support indicates a norm concerning teamwork. Allen and Kraft (1981) mention six principles that lead to productive work norms and a more satisfying work environment. All workers should have the six elements described below.

PRODUCTIVE WORK NORMS TEST

- *Involvement:* a say in setting their own work objectives and methods.
- *Clarity of organization and structure:* a clear job description and a clear role in the organization.
- *Feedback and information:* ongoing evaluation and recognition for their work and acknowledgment of their contribution to the overall organization.
- *Orientation and training:* the opportunity to obtain the skills and knowledge needed to do the job well.
- *Rewards:* positive recognition for accomplishments.
- *Supportive culture:* support from work colleagues.

Are these the norms in your organization? You can see the overlap of some of these areas with the organizational climate questionnaire (Table 6-2). The norms of the informal structure determine the work climate even more than the formal structure does.

Take time to reflect on these six areas in your health care system. What are some norms you see operating within your system in two of these areas? What is your contribution to maintaining one of these work norms? Realize that your contribution to keeping a norm may be "silent consent."

The organizational communication system is composed of upward and downward communication structures. Research shows that individuals communicate upward more easily than downward; this communication is designed to create an image of competency and capability in their position. As stress on a unit increases, communication often decreases and information is withheld. You, as a manager, need to see this as a warning sign.

Of the five types of information that move downward in an organization (Katz & Kahn, 1966) during stressful times, the predominant type is job instructions. The other four (job rationale; procedures and policies; feedback; and indoctrination of goals) support the nurse seeing the manager as someone other than a person "who tells me what to do." These four are the whys and wherefores of job instructions. If you are not also giving your staff these types of information, you are probably operating on overload. All five types are necessary for the nurse to have an organized systems approach to patient care.

Directing

A manager must direct the planned and organized nursing strategy. Directing involves four interrelated aspects: delegation, supervision, coordination, and control (Dimock, 1958).

Delegation is assigning tasks to people who possess the skill and competency necessary to carry out the task. Managers may choose not to delegate because holding someone accountable for their performance may involve disciplining. In "managing by objectives" (Odiorne, 1965, 1975), the staff is involved in planning objectives and in determining the direction of the objectives; thus they feel more responsible for their performance. In practice, management by objectives has failed many times because managers passed down the objectives instead of involving the staff. Management by objectives helps clarify the performance expected from each individual; this clarity facilitates delegation and disciplining.

Stress in the act of directing can be reduced by having clear objectives, policies supporting these objectives, and clear strategy. Clear job descriptions support individuals in knowing their responsibilities. Stress is reduced for the staff and for the manager if the act of directing is done efficiently and effectively.

Nurses at the manager level need to maintain a consistent objective and empathic stance. Promotion practices based on favoritism rather than clear, obtainable objectives produces a work unit filled with resentment. If the nurse manager is also unsympathetic, a stress-laden and dysfunctional work unit will result.

When managers delegate responsibilities, they are not only developing the management skills of the staff, they are also freeing themselves to deal with long-range planning. Once the duties are delegated, the staff needs sufficient latitude to determine the appropriate means to accomplish the task. Finding the balance between giving orders and allowing for a degree of professional freedom is the art of managing.

There are external and internal barriers to delegation. An external barrier is personnel who are not responsible in their task performance. If nurses fail to complete the budget or their patient care, they are not following through on the responsibilities accepted. This creates a lack of confidence in personnel and therefore the manager is under stress. An educator may have stress upon finding that students are not performing their tasks adequately.

Internal barriers range from lack of ability to delegate, to fear of criticism for mistakes in delegation. The manager's attitudes toward delegation play the major role in the quality and quantity of delegation. In order to minimize the risk taken in each delegation, the manager needs to consider the skill and competency necessary for the task. Delegation is meant to reduce stress not raise it.

To direct effectively, the manager must also supervise the "delegees." In supervising, the manager needs to support the staff in performing well. Most nurses are committed to giving quality patient care even in adverse situations. It is important in supervising not to let this commitment go unappreciated.

Supervising means guiding personnel to be most competent in their work. The type of guidance should be based on the individual staff member and the situation. Continuing educational opportunities and repeated feedback are necessary ingredients for effective supervision. Consistent, fair action by a supervisor supports the staff in honest upward communication without fear of reprisal. Ineffective supervising increases the staff nurses' stress levels.

Coordination is also an element in the process of directing. In learning to coordinate nursing activities for a patient, a student needs to be taught the importance of the interdependence of health personnel. The coordination necessary for patient tests or surgery is extensive. The con-

sequences of poor coordination cost the patients emotionally and finan-
cially. As the hospital system grows more complex coordination becomes
a key issue in patient care.

Some coordinating activities are used to prevent problems, while
others are used to resolve a particular problem. For example, both types
of coordinating activities are used by the operating room team and infection control team to deal with a patient with a streptococcal infection who
needs repeated surgery. Breakdowns in coordination raise stress levels
because they raise the level of uncertainty.

When coordination of activities fails, stress often results. For instance, when instructors do not coordinate their teaching activities in the
medical module, students are likely to become bored with the duplication
or confused over the lack of clarity. Staff nurses may experience the same
feelings when the x-ray and dietary departments fail to do their part in
the surgical preparation of a patient.

Controlling

The manager's job is also to control the planned, organized, and
directed strategies. The organizational philosophy determines the type
and the amount of control. The degree of control the manager exercises
needs to be congruent with the organizational policy and his or her own
supervisory ability; if not, the stress of role conflict ensues.

The manager exercises control in order to make sure that the actual
operations of the nursing staff conform to the planned operations; the
staff performance needs to be measured against established standards.
These standards are the basis for decisions concerning corrective action;
"without provision for action to correct deviations, the entire control
process becomes a pointless exercise" (Arndt & Huckabay, 1980).

Burned out administrators tend to assume authoritarian control:
"They tend to structure their administrative actions to promote their own
security . . . [They] obstruct with bureaucratic gibberish . . . [and] dog-
matic resignation . . . [and they] no longer engage in risk taking" (Veninga, 1979). Managers with these characteristics make for an organizational environment fraught with interpersonal stress and conflict.

Too little, as well as too much control harms working relationships.
A manager needs to decide what to be responsible for in relation to the
overall expected results. Effective leadership is situationally based. The
type and amount of control the manager typically takes depends on the
level of competence and skill of the staff. Taking too much or too little
control is stressful for all concerned.

Arndt and Huckabay (1980) divided the controlling function into
three aspects: preaction, concurrent, and feedback control methods. An

example of preaction is hiring a capable nursing staff. Concurrent control would be used to implement the planned rotation of ICU nurses. Quality control is a form of the feedback type of control. Plans may be redesigned as a result of this feedback.

Nurses experience stress if they are responsible for decisions over which they have no control. Frustration is the result of planning, organizing, and directing the students' learning and having insufficient control over the evaluation procedures. In both work situations and personal life, the sense of control reduces stress.

Look over the management skills listed in Table 6-6; in which do you see your greatest need for improvement? Make a list of those skills.

In which of these aspects of managing are you willing to make a commitment to increase your skills? List your first three action steps to make this commitment a realization.

WANDELT STUDY ON WORK CONDITIONS

A discussion of management's role in the prevention of burnout in nursing would not be complete without mention of some of the results from the Texas survey conducted by the School of Nursing at the University of Texas, Austin. Wandelt, Hales, Merwin, Olsson, Pierce, and Widdowson (1980) cite specific reasons for job dissatisfaction, including a lack of support by hospital and nursing service administrators. Administrators frequently sided with physicians in conflicts, leaving nursing unsupported.

Wandelt et al. (1980) also noted, "It is not the sheer labor of the work, it's the tension of not having a say over your own actions and not having confidence that patients are getting safe care that drives nurses out of the work force."

In Chapter 5 the focus was on nurses developing a plan to improve their work environment for the purpose of improving patient care; working in hospital conditions that make this difficult creates worry and frustrations. Leaders in nursing can play a role in creating desirable working conditions. The Wandelt study showed that most of the problems could be remedied without major expenses. Nursing administrators should make sure they get the administrative training they need. Administration has grown more complex and seniority will no longer make an adequate nursing director. As a role model and the nurses' liaison to hospital management, nurse managers need to continually improve their management skills. Managers in any large business or industry are expected to do so; if you are a manager, for your sake and for the sake of the nurses who work under you, please do so.

Some of the features of a hospital with desirable working conditions were quoted in *The American Nurse* ("Work Conditions," 1980). These

Table 6-6
MANAGEMENT SKILLS ASSESSMENT

Planning

Collecting and interpreting facts
Developing action plan forecasting the future
Implementing procedure for plan
Developing monitoring system and evaluation
Defining performance measures
Formalizing individual and organizational goals
Prioritizing goals
Assessing the organization's assets and liabilities
Assessing people and physical environment
Diagnosing communication problems
Weighing alternative solutions
Making clear, simple, and defined plans based on objectives
Creating stable and flexible plans
Assessing sociopolitical environment

Organizing

Grouping activities
Establishing relationships
Coordinating activities

Directing

Delineating authority and responsibility
Delegating responsibility
Decentralizing decision making (as possible)
Considering competence of the individual, information available, and impact of
    decision when delegating
Enforcing decision
Being aware of formal and informal structure
Being aware of social norms (especially communication)
Communicating in five types of downward communication
Supervising and guiding personnel
Coordinating personnel

Controlling

Carefully selecting and placing personnel
Limiting interruptions
Managing time effectively

and others listed in the study are useful as recommendations for prevention of burnout. You will notice some similarities between these recommendations and those of the National Commission on Nursing.

> A head nurse with a baccalaureate degree (or a master's degree) would have full responsibility on the unit for personnel, including hiring.
>
> All nursing care would be provided by registered nurses, with associate staff doing secretarial and other nonnursing related activities.
>
> Assigned staff would plan their own work schedules for days off, shifts, etc.
>
> Nurses on day and night shifts would have equal input into the total nursing care program.
>
> Inservice training would be planned so nurses could meet their own education needs.
>
> Pay differential would be provided for day and night shifts so enough nurses would choose nights, and day nurses would not have to rotate to other shifts.
>
> Collaboration among other units and hospitals would enable nurses to have a choice of opportunities to update skills.
>
> Salary increases would be tied to performance and recognition of good work.
>
> Nurses would have input into all policies affecting them, including nursing practice, patient care, and personnel benefits.
>
> Nurses would share planning for patient care with physicians and other health care administrators, and take part in decisions about patient discharge or movement to another care unit. ("Work Conditions," 1980, p. 19)

Use this list as one source of points you as a manager or educator need to consider in improving the working conditions of nurses.

In this chapter the role of management as the caretaker of the organizational climate was delineated. The first six chapters were designed to help you raise your awareness and gather information. At this point you are likely to be aware of a number of lifestyle and work-related issues you need to address. The purpose of the next chapter is to help you begin the process of change by increasing your understanding of your own change process.

7

How to Minimize Stress While Making Changes

CHANGE AS A STRESSOR

If there is one thing you can count on it is change. Change occurs on a cellular level and on a universal level continuously. We experience discomfort with change when it feels out of control. Changes that are out of our control are often sudden and imposed on us. Abrupt, sudden changes frighten us. We have trouble adapting our thinking and can become confused and overwhelmed by such changes. Remember your first "code" or an unexpected death, and you can see that the suddenness of these events played a major role in your stress reaction.

Changes imposed upon us without our imput into the process often trigger the fight side of the stress reaction. We become angry at the person imposing the change and may even sabotage the change. For example, the nursing Kardex format is changed and you had no say in the design process. You are likely to resist, at least initially, because the change lacked your early participation. Changing for someone else is always harder than changing because you yourself see a need to change.

The other aspect of change that affects your stress level is the significance of the change on the rest of your life. Your child or your spouse developing a chronic illness would have a profound impact on your life. A gradual erosion of your ego by a critical superior would also have far-reaching effects on your work and your personal life.

Changes not affecting you directly are often not seen as significant. Many people outside of Philadelphia may never have known about the teacher's strike in Fall 1981, which directly affected school nurses and indirectly affected businesses of all sorts. The level of significance of the change can only be determined by the person experiencing the change.

The significance of the change to an individual depends then on the impact of the change. Sudden, imposed changes that are significant are the kind that usually create a crisis in our lives—probably because these changes feel most out of our control. Extensive research with both humans and animals suggests that two related psychological factors can mediate an organism's responses to the stress of change: controllability and predictability (Krantz, 1980). Perceived control is defined as the felt ability to escape, avoid, and/or modify threatening stimuli (Averille, 1973). Predictability is the felt ability to anticipate a particular stimulus.

Increased predictability can help minimize the stress of making changes. If you can prepare for events they are less stressful when they occur and you are less anxious while you are awaiting them. The fear of the unknown is a potent stressor that needs reduction.

The information presented in this chapter can help increase your sense of the predictability and controllability of the process of change. Increasing your range of options can increase your sensed control. Maximizing your sense of control while making changes minimizes your stress.

Our degree of control over change is a question debated by more psychologists and spiritualists than I care to mention. However, one theme encountered frequently has particular relevance here—the wisdom to know the difference between what we can control and what we cannot control. When you are deciding to change something make sure it is realistically changeable, otherwise your efforts will be repeatedly frustrated. For instance, it is unrealistic to attempt to change your staff's negative attitude without changing your own.

To keep tension at a low level while you are effecting a change, you first must conduct an assessment of your present, future, and past relationship to change. In order to plan a change you must assess your present level of change and your anticipated future levels to decide if adding another change right now is beneficial or a hinderance to your stress management. In the first section of this chapter you will assess the effect of your present level of change upon your health. In the next section anticipated future changes, both in your control and not in your control, are considered. The questions are designed to help you evaluate your anticipated change environment for the future. The answers will help you plan any change you intend to make within the context of that environment.

In the third section your past handling of change is addressed with two questions: How have you handled change? How have you made changes? The purpose is to help you understand your typical response to change when you are not the originator of change, and also when you decide to change. Typical issues and skills that are involved in the change

Table 7-1
SOCIAL READJUSTMENT RATING SCALE

Life Event	Mean Value
1. Death of spouse	100
2. Divorce	73
3. Marital separation	65
4. Detention in jail or other institution	63
5. Death of a close family member	63
6. Major personal injury or illness	53
7. Marriage	50
8. Being fired at work	47
9. Marital reconciliation	45
10. Retirement from work	45
11. Major change in health or behavior of a family member	44
12. Pregnancy	40
13. Sexual difficulties	39
14. Gaining a new family member (e.g., through birth, adoption, oldster moving in, etc.)	39
15. Major business readjustment (e.g., merger, reorganization, bankruptcy, etc.)	39
16. Major change in financial state (e.g., much worse off or much better off than usual)	38
17. Death of a close friend	37
18. Change to a different line of work	36
19. Major change in the number of arguments with spouse (e.g., either a lot more or a lot less than usual regarding child rearing, personal habits, etc.)	35
20. Taking out a mortgage or loan for a major purchase (e.g., a home, business, etc.)	31
21. Foreclosure on a mortgage or loan	30
22. Major change in responsibilities at work (e.g., promotion, demotion, lateral transfer)	29
23. Son or daughter leaving home (e.g., marriage, attending college, etc.)	29
24. In-law troubles	29
25. Outstanding personal achievement	28
26. Wife beginning or ceasing work outside the home	26
27. Beginning or ceasing formal schooling	26
28. Major change in living conditions (e.g., building a new home, remodeling, deterioration of home or neighborhood)	25

29.	Revision of personal habits (e.g., dress, manners, association, etc.)	24
30.	Troubles with the boss	23
31.	Major change in working hours or conditions	20
32.	Change in residence	20
33.	Change to a new school	20
34.	Major change in usual type and/or amount of recreation	19
35.	Major change in church activities (e.g., a lot more or a lot less than usual)	19
36.	Major change in social activities (e.g., clubs, dancing, movies, visiting, etc.)	18
37.	Taking out a mortgage or loan for a lesser purchase (e.g., a car, television, freezer, etc.)	17
38.	Major change in sleeping habits (much more or less sleep, or change in part of day when asleep)	16
39.	Major change in number of family get-togethers (e.g., a lot more or a lot less than usual)	15
40.	Major change in eating habits (a lot more or a lot less food intake, or very different meal hours or surroundings)	15
41.	Vacation	13
42.	Christmas	12
43.	Minor violations of the law (e.g., traffic tickets, jaywalking, disturbing the peace, etc.)	11

Adapted from Holmes, T.H., & Rahe, R.H. The social readjustment rating scale. *Journal of Psychosomatic Research*, 1967, *11*, 213–218.

process are presented. Skills needed for the change process are examined in the last section. A self-assessment of your skills and suggestions for improvement are included.

PRESENT LEVEL OF CHANGE: EFFECTS ON PHYSICAL HEALTH

Before deciding upon a change, it is best to understand the stress your body and mind are presently coping with. In order to maintain changes at a tolerable level you have to know the impact of the ones you are presently experiencing. The scale presented in Table 7-1 is designed to help you see the impact of life events on your ability to cope. Holmes and Rahe (1967) investigated the effects of change upon our physical health and found a correlation between the changes a person experiences and the subsequent development of illness. They developed a scale containing 43 life event items with mean values reflecting the intensity of change. In Table 7-1, list the mean value of all the life events that have occurred in your life in the past year.

Add all the mean values you listed to find your total score. This score indicates the degree to which you are likely to get sick in the coming year. It does not indicate whether you will get sick; it measures the likelihood of your getting sick. A score of 300 or more indicates an 80 percent chance of illness, and a tendency toward multiple episodes; a score of 150–299 indicates a 50 percent chance of illness in the near future; and a score less than 150 indicates a 30 percent chance of illness in the near future. As you can see, the higher your level the less immune you are to bacteria, viruses, environmental pollutants, and people problems, and therefore the more likely it is you will have a physical, psychological, or behavioral illness. Your score is an indication of the likely effect of change upon your health.

After taking this test and reading this chapter on change, you may decide to spend your time and energy adjusting to the changes you circled in this index. You need to learn to adjust to changes you cannot control and direct changes you can control. Several studies that used this index led to relevant conclusions concerning the stress of change.

This index was used as a measure of health risk in two studies. Oskins (1979) found that 57 percent of 79 ICU RNs were at risk (scored over 150 in life changes). A similar risk may exist in other nursing populations. Bell (1977) examined the relationship between stressful life events, mental illness, and the wellness behavior in psychiatric and nonpsychiatric subjects. The psychiatric group experienced significantly more stressful life events. Persons with high change scores used more short-term coping methods than long-term methods; the healthier group used long-term coping methods. This study demonstrates the possible connection between these change events and psychiatric illness.

Studies assessing affective state and life events close to the development of cancer were done by Greene (1966) and LeShan and Worthington (1956). Their findings suggest that the loss of an intensely dependent relationship frequently occurs shortly before the clinical onset of cancer.

Two studies further illuminate the relationship between change and illness. Gatchel and Proctor (1976) demonstrated that subjects who did not know whether they could control a noise or did not know how to control the noise experienced a greater stress reaction than subjects in a clearly uncontrollable situation. Suls and Mullen (1981) assessed illness, perception of control, and desirability of real-life events. It appears that a life change must be perceived as *both* undesirable and not under personal control in order for it to have an effect upon illness; neither the undesirability of life change nor the lack of control over life change was sufficient in itself to result in illness.

This index is meant to help you make decisions concerning changes; it is not meant to scare you away from changes. In considering making a change you need to consider this index a variable, not make it your only guide for your decision. If your score was over 150 perhaps you should approach change with a degree of caution. What, if any, information modifies your concern over your score?

ANTICIPATED CHANGES

Consider anticipated changes that are not in your control. For instance, is your job in jeopardy or can you anticipate significant changes in your job within the next year? If you anticipate changes in your work, they will probably fall into one of the categories described below.

MAJOR CHANGES IN ORGANIZATION ASSESSMENT

- *Major reorganization:* merger with another hospital or university, or purchase by another organization; change in top administration; major policy or procedural shifts.
- *Change in the nursing process:* for clinicians, change from team to primary care; for managers, decentralization; for teachers, change in teaching style (individual to team) or teaching load.
- *New immediate boss:* consequent change in your own role (responsibilities, functions, relationships, perhaps increased role conflicts and role ambiguities with superiors, peers, and subordinates).
- *Job change:* change through promotion or relocation, perhaps requiring additional education or other preparation. Your answers to the following questions will directly influence your feelings concerning you new job: With my new job what will change? Will my authority (hiring and firing, disciplining, decision making) increase with my responsibility? With my increased responsibility will I have increased resources (people, supplies, equipment)? With my increased responsibility will I have increased rewards (money and benefits)?

Each of these categories is progressively more personal and more in your control. By anticipating these changes you can begin planning. Through planning change you feel more in control. Minimizing stress while making changes requires extensive planning and anticipation of Murphy's law in action.

Now consider anticipated changes that are in your control. In the next year what changes do you anticipate over which you have control? Make note of those items in Table 7-2.

Table 7-2
ANTICIPATED CHANGES IN YOUR CONTROL

Work life

Am I seeking a new job?

Am I seeking promotion?

Am I seeking education and experience necessary to do my job successfully and enjoyably?

Am I seeking the people skills (personal growth, courses, therapy) to communicate and relate at work and home?

Personal life

Am I moving?

Am I changing my primary relationship through marriage, separation, or divorce?

Am I changing relationships with my parents, children, or other significant family members?

Am I changing my relationship with any of my friends or significant others, such as mentors or religious leaders?

All these questions are designed to help you look at the changes you anticipate over which you have some control. If you are contemplating, designing, or presently seeking change in any of these areas then you need to determine the impact of that change upon you. Before you develop a change program in another area, you need to decide what changes you are already anticipating. List any changes you are planning to make in the next year. This information will help you plan change while minimizing stress.

To assess the potential effect of these changes you need to consider some of the mediating factors:

Magnitude:	loss of husband versus cousin; moving to a new city versus 10 miles
Unpredictability:	abrupt, sudden versus planned
Intensity:	all at once versus planned over time
Duration:	chronic, long-term effect of arthritis versus broken arm.

The more vigorous and severe the changes you anticipate the more taxed you are likely to be. The way you see these anticipated changes influences your response. As you reflect on the changes in your life considered in these first two sections, notice which ones will require you to adjust your coping system. Notice which ones could be altered by shifting your perception of the event.

PAST MANAGEMENT OF CHANGE

In order to make the process of change easier you must consider not only your present level of change and your anticipated changes, but also your past ability to handle change. At present this is your best predictor of how you will handle a new change. Your adeptness at managing change needs to be assessed on two planes. First, you can assess your ability to adapt to changes that have come because external or internal crisis conditions forced you (at least to some degree) to change your ideas, values, or behavior. How you handled these changes will provide you with information about how you generally deal with such changes. Some of the ways you handle stress actually increase your stress, while others lead to a reasonable adjustment to work or personal changes. Second, you can assess how you make planned changes. This involves assessing your cognitive processes of decision making, problem solving, and goal setting as well as values clarification, time management, and use of support resources.

It is important that you first understand your response to changes and then learn to know your general pattern in making changes. Later the skills required to support you in handling and making changes are examined. For now, begin to assess your need for these skills by viewing your style of managing change.

How Have You Handled Change?

The answer to this question depends on a number of factors. Basically, how you view a change, what you think about the change, and what coping behavior you institute determine your management of change.

Did you see the change coming or were you blind to it and therefore surprised by the change? Our 12 defense mechanisms (Freud, 1946) are part of our coping apparatus. When mechanisms such as denial, rationalization, and reaction formation are overused you become blind to your changing reality. A distortion of your vulnerability, "It won't happen to me," or a distortion of your capacity, "I can't go back to school" lead to blocks in coping with change. More often than not the rug is not pulled out from under you; the truth is you were not aware of the changes happening about you.

The reason you may be blind to certain changes is related to the response the change demands. If you determine in your mind that you cannot cope with certain changes you will either deny subsequent stimuli or their significance. This discounting mechanism of your mind serves to protect you from threats. If you see change in general as threatening, then you are likely to reduce your view of the world to avoid the threat of change. The wider your view of the system, the more successful your change strategy is likely to be. This open assessment response keeps your mind seeing and processing, not blind with fear or anger.

If you view change as a crisis rather than as an opportunity, your biological stress response is triggered. Your initial response is to fight or flee the change because you experience it as a threat. If you see the change as an opportunity, you become concerned with how to use it to your advantage. You may view the change as a chance to gain income, status, freedom of choice, or emotional stability, or as a chance to use your ability and knowledge; this approach often leads to handling change in a decisive manner. The question, "What can I learn from this change?" focuses on change as an opportunity. It is important for you to know your typical response pattern; changing this pattern begins with awareness of your fight or flight responses. Several patterns of behavior stem from the two feelings—anger and fear—that are associated with this response. The feeling of anger, associated with the fight response, originates because someone or something is not changing according to your desires. They may be changing or not changing, the issue is that the changing is not meeting your needs. Aggression toward the person who is suggesting or forcing changes is the behavioral result of handling the change with anger.

Less obvious aggressive techniques such as lateness, forgetting, giving misinformation, embarrassing someone, or being sexually provacative are ways to show anger at an imposed change. These passive-aggressive behaviors are the subtle sabotage methods that cost hospitals millions of dollars. They cost individuals personally, too, for close supportive relationships are impossible in the context of those behaviors.

Fear, the feeling component of the flight response, is a reaction to a threat to our physical or emotional security. Identifying which change situations are likely to trigger your fear response and which trigger your anger response is important in understanding how you handle change. You identified some in Chapter 3 (pp. 42–43). Your behavior motivated by fear hinders effective handling of most change. Most change is not physically threatening; it is ego threatening. If your ego security is threatened by fear of making a mistake or fear of failure, you are likely to flee or withdraw in situations in which action is appropriate. These fears could be preventing you from going back to school or taking a promotion.

Procrastination is covert resistance to change. When you are procrastinating you are neither openly saying no nor acting on the change. You are stalling or dragging your feet in the change process. If you procrastinate in response to changes, first recognize you are responding in a threatened manner. Handling change in this manner can become a dangerous coping habit. Procrastination creates more stress than it avoids (Knaus, 1979).

Identify your basic attitude toward change—opportunity or crisis. Are you usually caught off guard with changes? If so, what types catch you? If change is a crisis, then do you usually handle it through fighting or fleeing? List two changes you have handled well and two you have not handled well. Examining your style of making changes will shed light on your answers to these questions, for often unplanned change is viewed and handled as a crisis.

How Have You Made Changes?

By answering this question you will obtain a picture of how you generally decide on, prepare for, and act upon changes. Your past decision, preparation, and action habits are good predictors of your future handling of change; your awareness of these patterns is therefore important. By examining how you have changed past habits or handled situational problems you will understand that you already know how to change successfully.

Unfortunately, most people do not take the time for the analysis and the preparation involved in effective, planned change. If you are successful, you may believe it is because of luck or chance. Many of these times, however, you have gone through an unconscious change process.

The purpose of this discussion is to bring to your consciousness a model for change that is effective and involves minimal stress. Parts of this model will feel familiar to you; other aspects will seem new. Each aspect of the model is discussed in the next section on skills required for change.

To begin understanding how you have made changes, remember a change you made in your life that is recent enough for you to remember some of the details. Use this change as an example in the discussion of the process that follows.

The stimulus for that change was either external or internal. Someone or something in your environment forced you to take a look at yourself and your beliefs. This external feedback could come from a natural occurrence, such as a birth or a death, or from a shift in your relationships at home, work, or in your social world.

The internal stimulus is often a clash of values. Valuing yourself as an effective teacher and not doing a good job teaching because you are burned out creates the conflict that motivates change. When we do not live according to our values, our conscience troubles us in order to motivate us to align our behavior with our values.

Role conflicts are a good example of this internal clash of values. Assume you value being a good mother or father. You see spending time with your children as a measure of your being a good parent. A clash can occur when being an effective nurse takes time that you feel should be spent with your children. Stress reduction involves living within a framework of values. In any change process you need to make sure your desired change is aligned with your values, otherwise guilt and anxiety will ruin your plan. As you may remember, they are the consequences of not living according to your values.

The stimulus, whether external or internal, is a demand placed on the body or mind to change. The resulting stress is the body's or mind's effort to cope with this demand. You have made changes in order to cope with this stimulus.

Some stimuli have not been powerful enough to motivate you, while others have set you on fire. Disease is the body's way of saying you are not listening to its message stimuli. Signs and symptoms are messages warning that a change is necessary. The signs may be high turnover, poor-quality students, or headaches; all are warning stimuli.

Unfortunately, in our medical culture we are still disease and treatment oriented. If we were signs and prevention oriented we would pay more attention to the early warning stimuli. We really only change to prevent a loss or make a gain; we could cut our losses and make large gains in our stress management through this prevention orientation.

At whatever level you recognize this stimulus to change, you at some point decide to stop something and start something else. Deciding what, and then when, to stop are the second and third stages of the change process. These stages are so intertwined it is difficult at times to see them as separate.

In deciding what you will change you struggle with several alternatives for a period of time until you reach some conclusion as to the best plan of action. The decision to change motivates you to seek information, support and other necessary resources for successful change. Too often, people decide to initiate the change before adequate resources have been collected.

By making this change process conscious you can increase your proficiency in changing. Four components are necessary to achieve a successful change with minimal stress: (1) identifying the problem; (2) realizing that the problem is a significant one; (3) recognizing that the problem is solvable; and (4) finally, realizing that you have the capacity to solve the problem. These components help push you over the edge to change and support you in the change process. Without any one of these you are doomed to not using appropriate skills. These are the same aspects that were discussed earlier as discounts to the problem-solving process.

When these aspects of solving a problem are in your control, you are ready to initiate a change. In your problem solving process you reach a decision as to what your goal is and then begin to decide how to get it. Often this process has been active long before you actually verbalize or act on the decision.

A specific model of change is detailed in Chapter 8 to help you engage in an actual planned change. Three warnings are relevant to using any model of change; all three are related to the what and the when of changing.

First, failing to decide carefully what behaviors you will stop and what behaviors you will start leads to most failed behavior changes. The reason most people fail in their changes is that they fail to fill the void created by stopping a behavior, and the void soon becomes filled with old behavior. A decision such as "I will stop procrastinating" without a plan as to what you will do instead will not lead to the desired change.

Second, if the substitute is not balanced with what you gave up you are likely to lose the battle for change. Taking the time to figure out all the benefits of the change—your driving forces of change—can help you at those crucial times when you feel the tug of the old habit returning.

When you have not sufficiently decreased the forces blocking your change then you are making your change very stressful. To have to deal constantly with these resistances increases your tension, which often leads to a breakdown in motivation. Decreasing those forces that restrain you from reaching your goal eases the change process.

Take the time to write down how you met the criteria for the change model in your previous change example: (1) How did you fill the void created by stopping one behavior? (2) How did you balance the benefits of change to make them more powerful than what you gave up? (3) How did you reduce those forces restraining your change?

If you are to change, it makes sense to do it the easiest way. Changing the easiest way involves selecting a goal, deciding what to do to facilitate the change and remove blocks, and taking the appropriate action steps. This process is incomplete without intermittent evaluation. If evaluation is done only at the time of failure, the plan is doomed. Periodic evaluation is preventive maintenance for your plan. Were there set evaluation times and procedures for your example goal?

The final stage of preparing for action on your decided change involves organizing your time and resources. Whether your goal is to gain one hour of leisure time a day or to create productive staff meetings, you will need to use the four management functions to manage your time. Planning, organizing, directing, and controlling time are involved in both of these goals. Did you effectively use your time in your change example?

In identifying your resources, did you consider your internal and external resources? Internal sources such as your ability to be creative and disciplined may need to be tapped. External sources such as people, organizations, and actual physical supports should be gathered for use in the change process. Also identify people who will be an external hindrance to your change. Be creative in winning them over to your side or learn to get around their impedance.

How have you made changes? You have used your change example to answer this question by following the change process from stimulus to evaluation. In examining the general process you may have noticed you felt comfortable in using your resource of people, but found you had difficulty in controlling your time by saying no and setting limits. In the next section the skills mentioned in this section receive more attention. Even if you feel comfortable and successful in using some of the skills, I still suggest you read the section. The refresher will help you when you plan your actual change in Chapter 8.

SKILLS IMPORTANT FOR EFFECTIVE CHANGE

Even though these skills are often taken for granted, if you lack them or use them poorly, the process of change will be stressful. Often people notice these skills only when they are having trouble changing some aspect of their behavior or the behavior of others. A manager's job is to manage the changing environment by planning, organizing, and directing. The six skills covered in this section are all necessary to make changes with minimal stress; they are:

Values clarification
Goal setting
Decision making
Problem solving
Time management
Human resource management.

The discussion of each skill includes self-assessment and information on developing the skill.

Without these skills life can be very stressful. It is difficult to relax when you feel unable to plan or organize your personal or work life. Planning and organizing nursing care or lesson plans are important aspects of accomplishing goals. Planning a time for a meeting, organizing the people and the needed equipment, and finally conducting the meeting increases your work self-esteem.

Table 7-3
VALUES CLARIFICATION

1. Are you

    more Spring or Fall?
    more a paddle or a ping-pong ball?
    more a leader or a follower?
    more a placid lake or a tossing wave?
    more physical than mental?

    Rank order your response to the following questions.

2. How do you learn best?

    lectures
    workshops
    independent study

3. Which is most important in a leader?

    self-assurance
    people skills
    intelligence

4. Which would you rather have happen to you if you had bad breath?

    be told directly
    receive an anonymous note
    not be told

5. Which nurse would you choose to promote to head nurse?

    B.S.N. with 2 years of experience
    Diploma graduate with 5 years of experience
    A.D. with some management training

6. Your work benefit package is changing. Which would you like to see included?

    higher education benefits
    better medical coverage
    5 days off a year, called "well-being days"

Adapted from Simon, S.B., Howe, L.W., & Kirschenbaum, H. *Values clarification: A handbook or strategies for teachers and students.* New York: Hart, 1972.

Values Clarification

In order to help you know some of your values, do the exercises in Table 7-3. These questions allow you to focus on your lifestyle and professional value orientation. There are no right or wrong answers; the answers tell you where your values lie.

Your value system guides your personal and your nursing actions. When your values are in conflict with the values of the organization you experience stress from this conflict. Wandelt et al. (1980) concluded that when quality of care is compromised because of the work environment, nurses become dissatisfied. The nurses value quality patient care and a humanistic work environment. Not living and working within your values creates the symptom of tension. This tension can motivate you to change your behavior or your values.

Values are attitudes learned from the verbal and nonverbal messages of others. Those people who are most significant to you have the most influence upon the development of your value system. Your parents, teachers, and now your friends affect your personal and social values. Bosses, mentors, and colleagues have an important effect upon your work values (Buhler & Massarik, 1968; Kirschenbaum, 1973, 1975).

The decisions you make every day are based upon your conscious and unconscious attitudes and values. Most of the time you do not think of this in terms of values; rather, you think of these acts as simple or complex day-to-day decisions. You are confronted with more choices than were previous generations, and the many alternatives can be bewildering. Alternative choices become less confusing if your values are clear. Knowing what values you hold reduces conflict and confusion

There are seven requirements for clear values. They are not concerned with the content of your values, but with the process of valuing. This process involves the thoughts and behavior surrounding a value, not the outcome of the decision.

For a value to be clear, the following are necessary:

It must be freely chosen.
It must be distinguished from alternatives.
The choice must result from a thoughtful consideration of consequences.
You must have a good feeling about it.
You must have pride in it and a willingness to talk about it publicly.
It must be acted upon.
It must be part of the total pattern of your life.

The purpose of this discussion is to help you begin to see what important values you hold. As you do the various values clarification exercises that follow, you may wish to check these seven points to see if the value is a clear one.

Your values often lack clarity because the development of values is a lifelong process. There are two important questions to ask yourself: What do I treasure? What are my guidelines in life? Before you can effectively choose goals and make decisions you must know what you want and what you value.

To help you determine some of your personal values, consider the exercise shown in Figure 7-1. This may be the first time you have thought about some of these subjects, so take your time. Your answers are important reflections of your values. Remembering that values provide the framework for goal setting, you may want to consider these results in your goal planning in the next chapter.

Your values provide a framework for both your personal and professional goals. If you found in Table 7-3 that you are more a leader than a follower and that you learn best by independent study, your goal could be constructing your own personal leadership course from the readings listed in this book. Living according to your value system and working toward some of the 20 things you want to do before you die will do a lot to reduce stress caused by frustration.

To further clarify your values you may want to do more of the exercises in *Values Clarification* by Simon et al. (1972). Values clarification is a lifelong process and therefore involves changing in order to stay current with your environment and yourself.

Goal Setting

Goals provide the framework within which you manage your time to achieve your objectives. Values are the even larger framework within which you decide on your goals. A *goal,* according to *Webster's,* is the aim or the object end that one strives to obtain. Success is the progressive realization of your own predetermined, worthwhile goals.

Balanced goal planning involves six areas: spiritual, physical, social, mental, financial, and professional. Your life needs to be balanced with a variety of goals and steps to achieve these goals in each area. Your daily "to do" list is aimed at accomplishing these goals. The list you formulate daily guides you in reaching long-term goals.

Take time to write down three goals for each of the six areas. Make your goals realistic, specific, and phrased in the positive. Do not write "stop procrastinating"; write instead what you will do. An example of a possible goal in each of the areas is listed below:

Spiritual: To live according to my values
Physical: To weigh 135 pounds
Social: To have a satisfying and fulfilling marriage
Mental: To get my B.S.N. degree
Financial: To invest $500.00 in money market certificates
Professional: To publish an article on staff leadership in 1984

20 THINGS I WANT TO DO BEFORE I DIE	$	R	*	5	S/D	1–5
1.						
2.						
3.						
4.						
5.						
6.						
7.						
8.						
9.						
10.						
11.						
12.						
13.						
14.						
15.						
16.						
17.						
18.						
19.						
20.						

FIGURE 7-1. Next to the numbers in the left column, identify the following items on the chart:

1. and 2.	Places you want to go to
3.	Person you hope to meet
4. and 5.	Tasks you want to complete
6. and 7.	Two adventures you would like to have
8. and 9.	Two skills you would like to learn
10.	A skill you would like to improve
11.	A book you would like to read or reread
12.	Something you would like to learn
13. to 20.	Make your own: think of education, family, leisure, personal growth, career, and long-range goals

Code the right-hand columns according to the following:

Column 1:	$ if it costs significant money
Column 2:	R if it is realistic
Column 3:	* if it would be a shame if you did not
Column 4:	5 if you will achieve it in five years
Column 5:	S if you can make it happen;
	D if it depends on someone else
Column 6:	1–5 listing five most important items.

Adapted from Simon, S. B., Howe, L. W., & Kirschenbaum, H. *Values clarification: A handbook for practical strategies for teachers and students.* New York: A & W, 1972.

Your goal planning requires more thought than the few minutes you just spent. You will need to expand your list and prioritize. Begin by taking one of the goals you listed and make a more detailed step-by-step list. Each goal requires steps to success. List the action steps you will need to take to accomplish this goal. Then prioritize your list and you are ready to begin transferring some of the activities to your daily "to do" list.

Goal setting is a stress reducer because goals give you a sense of direction, a means to obtain desires, and a measure of success upon attainment. Goal setting involves creating a life map for you to follow. Change is here to stay, so you might as well take a major role in creating the changes in your life.

Motivation to change and seek these goals comes from belief that you will achieve your goals. If you believe you will not reach your goal then you will hardly put out the effort required. Success is the realization of your own predetermined goals. Success motivates more than any external benefit can.

Internal motivation sets the stage for taking charge, whereas external motivators of fear and incentives have many disadvantages. Internal motivation stems from the human drive for achievement and for self-fulfillment. Developing a prioritized, detailed set of goals allows you to direct your motivation.

Your goal setting will define a direction for your change program. Your decision-making and problem-solving abilities influence your goal setting for change. These two cognitive processes help you to plan, design, and carry out your goals (Meyer, 1976).

Decision Making and Problem Solving

Decision making involves some key components in order to be successful. Take the quiz in Table 7-4 to see how healthy your last decision was. Pick an important decision you have recently made and check your answers to the questions to determine your ranking on this skill.

If you answered "yes" to all these questions, your decision-making ability is very healthy. If some of your answers are "no," you will probably find reading this section helpful. Each of the issues raised in Table 7-4 is considered specifically below. As you read about each one, take time to reflect upon how that step affects your decision making. Note your assets and your present limitations.

1. Define the problem clearly. Many times after we have assessed the situation we have a list of problems that need to be solved. The second step is to prioritize the problems in order of resolution urgency. Select

Table 7-4
HOW HEALTHY WAS YOUR LAST DECISION?

1. Did you define the problem clearly?
2. Was your decision congruent with your goal?
3. Did you identify alternatives and consider their consequences?
4. Did you choose criteria to evaluate your alternatives?
5. Did you consider your values in deciding?
6. Did you consider your available resources?
7. Did you set a plan of action for your decisions?
8. Was an evaluation process part of your final plan?
9. Were you able to sort fact from emotions?

one problem at a time on which to focus your attention. Even if they seem overlapping, focus on only one.

What is the goal of solving this problem? The purpose of problem solving is some identified end. In making decisions you need to keep an eye on the goal. The problem may be infrequent suctioning of a patient with copious secretions. Remember the goal is a patent airway for the patient; suctioning is just one way to treat the problem. Focusing on the goal expands your thinking. Reducing the problem and goal to a single simple statement promotes focusing; wisdom is useless in decision making without clarity.

2. Set appropriate, realistic goals. Decisions need to be congruent with the overall goal plan to solve the problem. Deciding what your goals are for your life or your day and determining the priorities of these goals helps you organize your thinking. A written patient care plan prioritized with important objectives is an effective time and decision management tool. The same kind of written plan can be conceptualized for each problem you are solving.

Decisions are the link between goals and action. Most people do not spend enough time planning. Planning for achievement of goals allows for a clearer vision in choosing from alternative courses of action. In planning emergency procedures and standards of care the stress of immediate decisions is reduced. You are able to act on previously chosen "code" priorities, which frees your mind to focus on new incoming information.

3. Generate the alternatives. Just as values often provide the framework for alternatives, brainstorming can extend your list of options. Brainstorming allows you to go beyond what is readily apparent. Knowing all your options helps reduce the uncertainty that creates the worry and anxiety of the unknown.

Consider the consequences. In considering the alternatives what are the advantages and disadvantages of each? Choose some criteria to evaluate your choices. Practicality, desirability, preference, and adequacy could be one set of criteria. Saying no to working a double shift has consequences, just as saying yes does. It is important to recognize your alternatives, even though they may not be the most desirable. Weigh the consequences with a view to maximizing your self-esteem.

4. Evaluate your alternatives to narrow your choices. You need to evaluate each alternative in terms of your goal, values, and resources. These can be part of your criteria for evaluation. Once you have weeded out options that are not valuable, you need to check for similarities and differences among the options remaining. The question is, which alternative will bring you closer to your goal?

Can you combine some of your alternatives? For example, left with the choice to keep Mr. Jones in ICU for another day or transfer him to the floor, perhaps an alternative would be a half-way unit. Another alternative may be to have a senior student interested in doing a case study in cardiology patients assigned to Mr. Jones. Your needs as charge nurse for a responsible decision, the patient's need for closer watching, and the student's need for clinical experience all combine for the best alternative.

5. Define your values. Are your values your own or do they come directly from the mouth of your nursing instructor 10 years ago? Values help you decide the answers to the questions about yourself, others, and what is important. Your answers to these questions help you decide the kind of nurse you are and what your nursing priorities are. Knowing what is important helps you make well-informed decisions, and important values lay the groundwork.

6. Know your resources. Elicit the cooperation of others in actually helping you or in emotionally supporting your decision. Unless you want to collect, decide, and act on all information, you need to think of what decisions and activities you can delegate. Delegation or responsibility helps leave your mind free to analyze information at a higher decision level.

7. Develop an action plan. Often procrastination is the result of being overwhelmed by the complexity of the problem or the complexity of the solution. For instance, in deciding to create clinical case conferences every week, look at the smaller components: subject, people, time, and place. Looking at these smaller components allows you to decide on steps. Do not forget setting time limits—they create an urgency that motivates you.

8. Determine an evaluation plan. The decision you made yesterday for patient Squink is not necessarily going to hold today. Instead of looking for the book on the universal rules of nursing, you would do better to keep in mind monitoring circumstances. Determine your criteria for evaluation as well as your time intervals for evaluation. The evaluation process gives you the feedback you need to alter your choices.

9. Differentiate fact and fantasy. You need to base your decision on how reality presents itself, not on how you wish it could be. The decision to assign patient Farguan to Ms. Lyno, L.P.N. needs to be based on your assessed knowledge of her skills, not on your hope that she can handle the patient. On the other hand, do not forget to ask yourself how you feel about the alternatives you are evaluating. You may find that what you think is the best idea is emotionally uncomfortable for you. Being uncomfortable with your decision is not necessarily a criterion for rejecting the decision.

In dealing with facts and fantasies, determine what is under your control. Your feelings, attitudes, and expectations are under your control. Social forces such as high turnover or Dr. Hard-to-get-along-with working at your hospital are forces of the general climate. Remember the importance of the wisdom to know what you need to accept and what you can change.

Your sense of well-being is a result of the decisions you make. Your decisions guide your professional life as a nurse with your patients and with your peers. Decision making is a skill; practice the skill by making up your mind to consider these guidelines for your next decision.

If after reading this material on decision making you feel you need better decision-making skills in your personal or professional life, consult the books by Arnold (1978), Bailey (1975), and Miller (1978). These books can help guide you in learning decision-making skills. However, since decision making is a skill, the best way to learn is through practice. Instead of "passing the buck," what is one decision you can make today that will reduce your stress?

After examining these various aspects of decision making, you can begin to see that problem solving is an exercise in decision making. A large part of your problem-solving ability is your attitude about problems and decisions. If you see yourself as a person unable to make decisions and as someone who thinks problems lack solutions, then you are blocking your progress in these skills. This attitude becomes a self-fulfilling prophesy after a time. Being a better problem solver begins with a belief that you can solve the problem with the appropriate help.

Collaborative problem solving was discussed in Chapter 5; the success of problem solving depends upon using this method and also on not falling into certain traps. The four traps that seem most often to catch people involve the handling of emotions, undiscovered hidden agendas which sabotage, lack of clarity around details, and lack of follow-up.

When you engage in problem solving you are dealing with your belief system and your emotions. Your emotions need attending to as well as your rational thoughts. Many times you can hear people say, "I know it is not rational, but I feel angry." Feelings that have not been dealt with are often the source for hidden agendas. Problem solving is hindered by these emotional barriers. If you notice that you are not progressing toward a solution at the pace you think appropriate, check for hidden agendas and hidden emotions.

If you do not like details, then you need to have someone involved in your problem-solving procedure who does. Too often this lack of attention to detail creates more conflict as the solution fails to materialize. Comments such as "These solutions do not work," are often a result of not attending to implementation details.

Finally, the lack of follow-through on solutions can create an atmosphere of distrust. People often interpret this behavior as indicative of a lack of caring, but it is most often a result of poor planning of the checkpoints in the evaluation process. If specific plans are not made, then other priorities can easily replace the action steps needed for the problem solution.

To solve problems effectively you must go through certain steps. This step-by-step process affords you the opportunity to see what areas of problem solving are most difficult for you. By considering the areas just discussed and by referring back to the section on collaborative problem solving in Chapter 5, you can assess what steps you need to pay special attention to in your process. Creating change is equivalent to solving problems. If you begin changing some of your stress components, you are solving your health problems.

Stress is often the result of somebody's faulty decision making or a result of your own poor problem solving. For example, your boss may be trying out a new evaluation system without proper education of the staff. The staff then feels scared or angry at not being educated. In this example a faulty decision on planning was made by your boss. You try to solve your overweight problem with the latest fad diet. This is another example of poor decision making. With this solution you will probably join the ranks of the other 60 percent of dieters who cannot keep the weight off.

Once you cease to look outside yourself for someone to solve your problems, you begin to become a free agent. Building an internal support system prevents the stresses of disorganization and poor planning. You are free when you no longer blame anyone for your happiness, but instead use your skill of problem solving to take charge of your life.

In using both decision making and problem solving skills you will be managing time and resources. Your time management involves you deciding on your approach to the problem. Managing people is usually involved in directing the solutions to time management problems. Time management is a necessary component in designing a change program.

Table 7-5
TIME WASTERS

Self-Imposed	System Imposed
No planning	Telephone
Socializing	Visitors
Preoccupation	Meetings
Lack of (or poor) delegation	Delays
Attempting too much	Interruptions
Involved in details	Poor communication
Unable to say no	Waiting for decision
Lack self-discipline	Mechanical failure
Wrong choice of priorities	Mistakes (other)
Procrastination	Secretary ineffective
Interruptions	Reverse delegation
Mistakes (your own)	Problem not clear
Failure to listen	Lack policies
Over control	Lack authority
Fear of offending	Understaffed
Unrealistic time estimates	Overstaffed
Unable to terminate visits	Different value system
Failure to anticipate	Lack of feedback
Goals not clearly defined	Role not clear
Slow reader	Low priority memos
Emotional upset	Shifting priorities

Reprinted from Hobbs, C. R. *Insight on time management.* Charles R. Hobbs Corporation, Salt Lake City, Utah: 1979. With permission.

Time Management

Managing your time is a way to prevent stress. If you feel you are always behind schedule, can never get caught up, or just cannot seem to get things done, then you need to learn to manage your time. Take the short quiz in Table 7-5 to identify those items that are time wasters for you.

From Table 7-5, select the five key ways you waste time and list them. Prioritize the list to locate the most troublesome problems of the five. Set a goal to reduce or eliminate the most vital problem. Write down the first action step you need to begin, and also when you will do the step. Then carry out your goal.

Time management requires you to examine the four areas of management—planning, organizing, directing, and controlling. For instance, in the area of planning, you need to establish a daily time to construct a prioritized "to do" list for the next day. Each evening or morning construct a schedule of the day's tasks, rating each one with a priority of 1 (vital), 2 (important), or 3 (of limited value).

Effective time management requires that your daily "to do" list is based on the most important activities required to perform the job you want to accomplish and that it is based in reality. Beginners in time management often construct "to do" lists that look like they are preparing for the week instead of the day. For work, the high-priority activities are the ones you get paid to do and against which your performance is measured.

Daily planning for emergencies requires you leave some spaces in your schedule for situations that require your immediate attention. Make sure before you note this emergency on your list that it is a true emergency by asking yourself these questions: Am I the only person who can extinguish this fire? If not, who else can? If the fire is left until tomorrow, is it likely to burn out, or spread? Make sure this is a real emergency and not your ego talking.

Organizing in time management means prioritizing and grouping activities. If you are caring for a patient with a recent myocardial infarction you would prioritize your care and then decide what aspects of the care could be grouped together. This applies equally to designing a lecture or deciding on continuing education needs.

Organizing your time, space, and paperwork can do a lot to help you function effectively. If you develop you own individual way of ordering your paperwork, rooms, closets, drawers, and daily activities, you will spend less time searching and have more time for doing. Giving up your rebellious ways against your parents' stance on order is often not as easy as you may have thought. Learning that freedom, not entrapment, comes from order is an important lesson.

Winston (1978) points out that the key to straightening things out is to know your organizing principle. This principle is based on the idea that any practical system has a central core around which all other components group themselves. First, you need to determine the focal point of your organizing principle. For example, if your organizing principle is status you will organize your life to reflect your status. The way you dress, where you live, the hospital or university you work for, all can reflect your need for status. If you organize around defiance of authority, then your choice might be just one form of rebellion. Other organizing principles could be achievement, security, or power.

Take time to reflect upon the central core around which you organize your life. This central principle determines how you structure your time, space, and maybe even your relationships. Your organizing principles reflect your values. If you value achievements you are likely to organize your time to obtain achievements and decorate your space with diplomas,

Table 7-6
HOW ORGANIZED ARE YOU?

1. Do you often misplace keys, glasses, gloves, handbags, correspondence, or other items?
2. Have you overlooked birthdays, appointments, or some specific date you wanted to acknowledge?
3. Do you find crisis situations arising because you "forgot" to do or get something?
4. Do you spend more than ten minutes trying to locate an article, a bill, or another item that you know "had to be right here"?
5. Have you ever "lost" something in your house only to have it reappear after several months?
6. Do you have stacks of unanswered correspondence, unfiled receipes, and unread magazines?
7. Are you frequently late for appointments, commitments, or other activities?
8. Do you have piles of items scattered around the house, in the basement, and in the garage waiting to be put away?
9. Do you feel that having more space is all that you really need to solve all of your storage problems?
10. Do you want to organize things but are turned off when you realize how much there is and you do not know where to start?
11. Do you usually feel that you haven't accomplished as much as you had hoped to before the day ended?
12. Are your frequently used items in hard to reach or out of the way places in your kitchen, bathroom, etc.?
13. Do you have to clear things out of the way before you can sit down to relax, visit, or work?

How to score
Score 1 point for "yes" answers only. If your total score is:

    1–3,   you are in good shape;
    4–6,   disorganization is causing stress in your life;
    7–9,   disorganization is interfering with your life;
    10–14, you need to take immediate action to get organized.

Adapted from John, D. *Time, space and paper management.* Philadelphia: Dorothy John & Associates, 1981.

certificates, trophies, or other symbols of achievement. Your relationships with your colleagues may be taxed at times because they see you as highly competitive. Take time to understand how your values or your organizing principles guide your time, space, and people organization.

First you need to understand where your organization problem lies, since most people are not disorganized in all areas of life. Define the problem by completing the questionnaire in Table 7-6. By assessing your

Table 7-7
STEPS IN DELEGATION

1. Select the people who have the ability to do the job.
2. See that they clearly understand what you expect.
3. Let them know you sincerely believe in their ability to carry out the task.
4. Secure a commitment that they will follow through.
5. Negotiate a deadline.
6. Provide latitude for them to use their own imagination and initiative.
7. Let them know in the beginning you are going to follow-up, and do it.
8. Do not do the job for them.
9. Reward them commensurately with the results they produce.

Reprinted from Hobbs, C. R. *Insight on time management*. Salt Lake City, Utah: Charles R. Hobbs Corporation, 1979. With permission.

personal level of organization you will be better able to see what areas are raising your stress level. List three key problems from those you just identified.

If being more organized would reduce the stress in your life, take the list of problems you identified and *Getting Organized* by Winston (1978) and begin. Getting organized will allow you to handle surprise situations more efficiently and effectively. Think of how great it would feel to be organized at home and in the office. Additional readings include those by Berman (1977), Kaltman (1971), Liman (1977), Skelsey (1970), and Tennov, (1977).

Directing to solve your time management problem involves delegation. Getting things done by people is a way you can triple your daily accomplishments. Follow-up on your delegated tasks takes less time than doing the project. Think of two activities you can delegate and to whom.

Delegating is the one aspect of time management that many altruistic helper types need the most help in changing. Too often they overburden themselves with tasks they feel they do not have the right to delegate. The stress of taking on activities that repeatedly put you out of your comfort zone will cost you more than the price of delegation. (If you could not think of two tasks to delegate, try again!)

Delegation is a process, not an end. The steps in delegation and some ideas to keep in mind while delegating are listed in Table 7-7.

Remember that if you have not been delegating to your staff and/or family you have to go through an adjustment period. They may be unhappy and respond negatively to your delegating; after all, it may require them to do more work. However, remember your goal is not to win the Popularity or the Martyr of the Year Award. Your goal is to take care of yourself while taking care of others.

The final aspect of time management is control. Decreasing distractions and interruptions will allow you to experience more control over your time. Saying no to people helps you take charge of your time. Remove yourself from your distractions when possible and eliminate unnecessary interruptions.

Start with the planning and work your way through to controlling time, examining the ways you would improve your time management. Lakein (1973), in *How to Get Control of Your Time and Your Life,* provides time management principles and practical suggestions. Armed with self-awareness of your time management problems, the advice in Laekin's book, and your commitment to reduce your time pressure stress, you can begin to manage time successfully.

Human Resource Management

Like time management, the management of people is a key to any change process. Whether your change process directly or indirectly involves people, your change will affect others. How you manage to help others in the change process will play a large role in the success or failure of your work or personal goal.

Delegation of your work is but a small part of managing the change process. Delegating decision making to the lowest level possible increases your children's, staff's, or student's involvement in changes that affect them. The more involved they are, the more motivated they will be to carry out their roles for the change.

Gain as much support for your change as possible. To gain the support of people for a change you desire you need to facilitate their seeing the benefits of the change for them; they may resist the change if you do not. Your planning for change must include ways to gather people's support for the change.

A good salesperson will always tell you the two keys to selling are belief in your product and convincing people of the benefits of your product. In other words, believe in your change and share with others the benefits you see in the change for them. Secret change plans, once shared, create either surprised or angry, shocked responses. You, as a manager of your household or your work unit, want to minimize others' stress responses to your changes. Involving people in your change project early in the process will promote support instead of shocked fight or flight responses.

For example, you want to change the orientation program for new graduates. You want to elicit support and faculty from the local university, which is the source of most graduates. How can you convince the university faculty that it would benefit them to be involved? In managing a change such as this, having them involved from the very beginning is the key.

A second example points to the importance of knowing who you can count on for support and who will hinder your change. A director of a nursing school decided she wanted to incorporate students' evaluations as part of the faculty evaluation process. She expected support from the faculty and hindrance from students, for they would have to do more evaluation of faculty. In fact she got the reverse. Rather than imposing this method of evaluation upon the faculty, a better approach would have been to involve the faculty in the research for alternative evaluation processes.

In looking for support be aware of how you can give support to others. People do remember your helping hand. They are more inclined to help if they have at least a rudimentary relationship with you. Managing people involves an exchange of support; otherwise one individual begins to feel used.

If you see yourself as having difficulty dealing with people to get the kind of support you would like, take a long look at your human relationship skills. Your communication, listening, asserting, and conflict resolution skills are all part of interpersonal relationships. Read *People Skills* by Bolton (1979) if you have a strong desire to improve your interpersonal relationships and are willing to experiment with approaches to communication. Improving your approach to people will help you gather the support you need in mastering a change.

In the first seven chapters you have been given tools to assess your stress level and to assess your level of skill in various areas. In order to carry on with some of the techniques suggested you will have to begin to change some health and lifestyle habits. Whatever goals you have made for yourself, you will need to involve yourself in a change process. In Chapter 8 you will focus on the process of change. You will begin to see how to identify the change you desire and take that change step by step to completion. Using the model presented will allow you to make changes with minimal stress.

8

Planning Your Own Program for Reducing Stress

ASSESSMENT: THE FIRST STEP IN CHANGE

Throughout this book you have become aware of aspects of yourself and your environment that contribute to your stress level. You have learned what habits you have that foster the development of signs and symptoms of stress, or possibly even a stress-related disease. By now, you know what you are doing or not doing that moves you in the direction of illness. You also have learned some skills that can reverse your path and send you instead toward high-level wellness. In each of the first seven chapters you were invited to look at how you presently conduct your life. Each was designed to raise your level of awareness about how you handle stress.

In order to change how you deal with stress you first need to be aware a change is necessary, and second to have options. Some options for changing your unhealthy habits have been presented. Other recommended resources can be found in each chapter. It is now time to think about planning your own change program for reducing stress.

Based on the wellness concept of self-responsibility, this chapter is a guide for you to take responsibility for managing your stress. You begin by tuning into your own inner patterns—emotional and physical—and recognizing the signals your body is giving you. Take time to go back over the preceding chapters and identify the signals of stress that your body is sending. Identify your stress-producing habits in each chapter.

For example, in reviewing Chapter 2 you may list too much sugar in your diet, no consistent exercise, and not enough alone time. In Chapter 4 you may list your perfectionistic tendency, and in Chapter 7 you may have found you have poor time management skills. You will list all these items in the restraining column of your personal assessment, described below. They are preventing you from maximum health. Also review your strengths, such as balanced diet (Chapter 2), no drugs (Chapter 3), and supportive work group (Chapter 5). It is essential that you know your strengths when you design your change process. Realizing you are the expert about you will foster your taking responsibility for your health.

Taking responsibility for reducing your stress involves choices. First determine through assessment what choices you have been making. The topics considered in the first seven chapters are listed below:

1. Introduction
2. Physical
3. Psychological
4. Behavioral
5. Work
6. Management's role
7. Change

Make a list with two columns, and as you review each chapter list your restraining forces, or liabilities, in the first column and your driving forces, or strengths, in the second. To help you in this assessment process, all the assessments and exercises you have done are listed after the Table of Contents at the front of the book. Taking time to do a proper assessment will assist you greatly in making your change successful. There is nothing like a black and white view of your present choices to help you determine your stress reduction goals.

As you read over the list you could be feeling anything from despair to excitement. Fear not, this is the first step toward change. Assessment can be painful because it points out your health and environment supports and liabilities. A larger list of strengths is possible by taking one liability and beginning to plan a change.

Through your personal assessment you have identified your stress producers and aspects of your life that can help you modify your stress. Your list is a picture of the sources of stress and a picture of skills, people, activities, etc., that facilitate you in keeping your stress within your comfort zone. The tell-tale signs and symptoms of stress take on more meaning when you see the whole picture.

Awareness of the problem is the first step in the change process. Defining the problem is the first step in the problem-solving process. The next step is identifying what particular problem you would like to work on first. The rest of this chapter is designed to guide you through the change process with whatever goal you choose.

The model of change used here is based in part on a personal growth group model of change formulated by Wheelan (1978). The model is based on current psychological and social theories and research and can also be used by individuals choosing to initiate a change process. The change process is as follows:

1. Goal identification and specification
2. Determination of the internal and external factors that contribute to the maintenance of the unsatisfactory behavior pattern
3. Development of a personal change strategy
4. Implementation and monitoring of the change strategy

GOAL IDENTIFICATION AND SPECIFICATION: WHERE DO I START?

Targeting a specific and attainable goal is the first step. Once you have decided to change you have set the wheels of change in motion. Setting goals that support this decision will make the decision a reality. The material presented in this section can help you gain clarity on what problem to tackle first and how to set realistic steps to gain control over the change process.

In identifying and specifying your change goal you need to consider four factors. First, the change you want must feel important to you. You need to feel that choosing this goal from your assessment list is important and that it has a high priority. This will help give you the motivation to change this negative stress management habit. The sense of motivation—some inner drive and intention—will make the other steps in the process seem less arduous.

What change would spur you on to greater health, satisfaction, or success? What do you want that probably money cannot buy? What change in your lifestyle, in your way of relating to others, or in your personality patterns would help you manage your stresses more effectively? Reflect for a few minutes. Write down your change goal. Word the goal in the positive. For instance, instead of "stop procrastinating," state "complete projects I begin." "Weighing 135 pounds" is more positively motivating than "losing 30 pounds." Word your goal to focus on what you want to accomplish, not on what you want to get rid of by changing.

Second, your identified goal should have personal meaning to you. Changing for someone else is doomed to failure. You need to be convinced of the benefits of changing. However, first make your goal statement in the positive and as specific as possible.

Specificity is the third factor in goal setting and achievement. Vague, general goals fail to motivate because they do not provide a clear image of what you want to accomplish. "Beginning an exercise program" may be a physical strategy to reduce stress; "to ride my bicycle three times a week for 30 minutes, with my pulse between 21 and 26 beats for 10 seconds," is a clear, specific goal.

Take your goal and make it specific. A few examples may be helpful: "To spend one evening a week in school (with my husband/working with community center)." "To take three continuing education courses in management skills this year." "To develop a support group of nurses in my hospital." All of these examples are action oriented toward a specific end. Further specificity is necessary, e.g., deciding which courses to take. The goal could be as specific as "I will take Psych 406, Theories of Personality, on Wednesday nights in the Fall semester." The more specific the goal, the easier it is to assess your progress.

In setting your specific goals it is important never to lose sight of your purpose and major goals. The importance of this is best illustrated by a story a nurse told me. She had decided to go back to school, and therefore she started taking courses. She had no degree goal in mind, she just wanted to take some courses. During this time she was in line for promotion for a head nurse position. Unfortunately, she was unable to get the position because the rule for over one year had been that a management position requires a B.S.N. She had the college hours, but her courses did not satisfy the requirements for a B.S.N. The hard lesson she learned was that short-term goal consideration needs to be done in the framework of long-term goals.

Write the specific goal that you will use to follow the change process in the remainder of this book. Reflect, and write your choice of change goal as clearly as you can. Whenever your goal is referred to in the following sections this is the goal you will remember. Perhaps you will further clarify it as you continue; if so, rewrite your goal.

Finally, sharing your goal with two other people to whom you are close will help you in the clarification and implementation process. This helps you begin to gather your resources for a supportive change environment. More on the role of their feedback and your sharing will follow. For now, list two people with whom you will share your goal and later your progress in attaining the goal. With these individuals, explore your feelings about this goal, discuss your fears and resistance to change, discuss plans to neutralize negative environmental forces, and assess the realistic and unrealistic expectations of yourself. All this processing helps to further clarify your goal. By openly discussing your goal and change process you will maintain motivation and foster commitment to your goal.

DETERMINATION OF INTERNAL AND EXTERNAL
FACTORS THAT MAINTAIN BEHAVIOR
PATTERNS

Using forced field analysis (Lewin, 1951), as you did in your personal assessment earlier in this chapter, you can develop a change strategy for your specific goal. To use this method you first identify what forces exist that restrain you from making efforts to change, and then you develop a strategy to reduce the potency of these forces. Identifying and increasing facilitating forces that support your change is just as important as identifying and decreasing the restraining forces.

Identifying Restraining Forces

The first question to ask yourself is, "What external factors in my life hinder me from reaching my goal?" Specifically, what people (spouse, friends, children, colleagues, boss, etc.) are involved in preventing you from obtaining your goal and how are they hindering you? What environmental factors, such as lack of privacy, hectic pace of work unit, and financial and community factors make it difficult to reach your goal? Think of your physical and people environment and identify as many external factors as possible that contribute to your maintaining your old habit. Reflect, and then list these factors.

These factors probably include some time wasters such as interruptions, mistakes of others, understaffing, mechanical failures, reverse delegation, and unclear role differentiation. For instance, you may have a goal of being a better manager by appropriately delegating responsibility to subordinates. A restraining external force could be an ineffective ward secretary. A boss could contribute to restraining this goal by poor communication and unclear policies. Reflect once more and see if you can add to your list of external forces that hinder you from reaching your goal.

Internal forces play a powerful role in preventing change. Some possible internal forces that restrain change are lack of self-discipline, fear of offending, unrealistic time estimates, inability to say no, and overcontrol. Procrastination and perfectionism are often partners as restraining forces. The question to answer is, "What internal thoughts and behavior patterns contribute to my maintaining my habit and not reaching my goal?" "How do I stop myself from reaching my goal?" Reflect, and then list these internal factors.

This list is important in helping you see where you need to reorganize your thinking and to redirect your action. Internal restraining factors, once reduced, free your mind to work toward accomplishing your goal. Both the internal and external restraining factors you listed are key aspects of your life you need to address to remove your blocks to change.

The next step is to select the most potent forces from these two lists and develop ways to eliminate or reduce their effect on your change goal. For instance, you have a chocolate craving every day at 3:00 p.m., and this internal force is one factor restraining you from losing 10 pounds. In this step you decide how you will deal with this factor by reducing its force. One solution could be providing another source of natural stimulation, such as sugar in fruit. Perhaps you would not have the craving if you ate a lunch with protein sources. Maybe exercising after work and treating yourself with something less costly to your waistline would be solutions.

In order to overcome the effects of some of the restraining forces you identify you may need to learn new skills. For example, perhaps you are a slow reader and you see this as a block to your success in school. Learning the skill of speed reading would be a step that could reduce your hesitancy to return to school.

Take time to list your most potent restraining forces. For each one, list ways to reduce the potency of its restraint achieving on your goal. Each restraining force is a roadblock to your change. Identify solutions to get rid of or reduce the power of the negative force.

Reflect upon your list of restraining forces and prioritize your determined actions for reducing their effects. Number them in the order in which you will put them into action. In the third stage you will use these prioritized actions to create a strategy.

Identifying Facilitating Forces

To support your success in this process, identify the forces that already exist and then take action to increase their potency. Both restraining and facilitating forces act on change.

Focus on both external and internal facilitators of change: What people can you count on for support, and how? What external environmental factors support you changing? What thoughts, behaviors, and skills do you already have that facilitate you changing? Look at past accomplishments; what facilitated you changing? What support do you need in order to maintain the change? Use these answers to help you answer the next question. What forces are driving you to make this change to reach your goal? List both internal and external forces. Next list your key driving forces for change and ways to increase their effect. Two examples of identifying the driving forces for effective educational programs follow. In one case the nurse educator's goal was to have the class involved in the presentation of the course. A driving force for this change was a resolution presented by the student body to the administration requesting more involvement in their educational process. She increased the force of this resolution by introducing her intended change in a resolution form to the students. The analogy was obvious.

In the second case an inservice director's goal was to convince the administration that more inservice educators were needed. One of the driving forces for this change was the results of a hospital survey. The survey showed that 85 percent of the RN staff felt their continuing education needs were not being met. She brought these results, a two-month time log of her activities, and a list of the educational needs of the staff to the attention of the director; as a result, the decision was made to hire two more educators over the next year.

Your own success story depends on you first identifying your restraining and driving forces of change and then finding ways to decrease the restraining and increase the driving forces. The next step is to develop a change strategy.

DEVELOPMENT OF A PERSONAL CHANGE STRATEGY

The third step in achieving a goal is to develop a change strategy. This strategy includes organizing your time and your resources. Your success depends on developing an effective strategy.

Time Management

Consider the four aspects of time management in relation to your goal; their importance in goal achievement is obvious. Planning, organizing, directing, and controlling your time all involve strategy. They are also relevant to gathering and allocating resources. You have already decided what needs to be done and prioritized your actions. You have a "to do" list that now needs to be further broken down to specifics with deadlines attached. In your daily "to do" list you should include at least one action that supports you reaching your stated goal. This helps keep the goal before you, acting as a motivator.

List five items that could appear on your "to do" list. These items are ways that either increase your driving forces or decrease your restraining forces. Make them specific enough so that you can begin action immediately. Next to each one write your deadline for completion. These actions are part of your plans for change.

Next organize these actions into components or groups. For instance, perhaps three of the actions involve assertiveness skills and the other two require management skills. Your strategy would then involve organizing your time to include an assertiveness course and management training. What skills will you need to reach your goals?

Directing your actions for the most effective time management often involves delegation. Ask yourself two questions: "What am I now doing that I or anyone else need not do?" "What am I now doing that someone else can do?" List your responses and the people to whom you will delegate the responsibilities. Remember the purpose of delegating is to help you achieve your goal. There is always something you could delegate if you really thought about using your time effectively to reach your goal. Nurses too often are blind to their resources because they are in the habit of doing it themselves. The burden is always easier when shared. Make sure your program for reducing stress involves some delegation.

The fourth aspect of time management is also important to goal achievement. Controlling your time through eliminating interruptions and saying no adds relaxation and more hours of personal time for yourself. How could you take control of your time to facilitate your goal? What would you be doing differently if you put yourself in charge of planning, directing, and organizing your time? Write down your answers to these questions.

You have now considered the role of each of the four aspects of time management in managing your time to achieve your stress reduction goal. List these key elements in your strategy for change. You can add to this list by briefly reviewing other strategies presented in this book. Physical, psychological, and behavioral as well as work strategies are all potentially useful in developing your overall strategy. Some methods are more relevant to your goal. Take time to see if any will further facilitate your change. Reflect upon the possibilities briefly reviewed below.

Brief Review of Strategies

The physical strategies for stress reduction (Chapter 2) involve actions that increase the body's adaptability to stress. The synergistic wellness triad of exercise, relaxation, and nutrition probably deserves some priority in your change strategy. Perhaps reducing coffee consumption would be a nutritional boost to achieving relaxation. Exercise would also promote relaxation by ridding the body of toxic chemicals and producing endorphins, which promote a feeling of well-being.

The psychological strategies for stress reduction (Chapter 3) include changing internal thought patterns that lead to stress and improving communication skills to change relationships. A brief review of Chapter 3 could prove useful in reducing restraining forces, such as guilt and perfectionism, and in increasing facilitating forces, such as getting recognition and developing a sense of humor.

Behavioral addictions are often potent restraining forces. Using specific strategies (Chapter 4) for each of the addictions will help decrease their effect on your change process. For instance, the effects of nutrition and the environment on the thinking process are just beginning to be understood; in reviewing the strategies for changing your nutrition you could add some key elements to your overall goal strategy.

Using your resources for ongoing support is mentioned a number of times throughout the book. Perhaps increasing your technical support system at work could help you be a more effective manager. By so doing you could get the feedback you need to help you identify issues and to support your change.

For specific work changes (Chapter 5) you could learn collaborative problem solving to help reduce the tension in your work unit. Perhaps you could clarify your role to your students or subordinates to decrease the stress of trying to function as a clinician-manager-teacher. Perhaps learning some new technical skill would decrease your stress.

In Chapter 6 you may have learned that management's goals are not clear to you and this ambiguity creates stress for you. You could seek clarification of the goals and perhaps establish a process whereby you are more involved in their formulation. Whatever your goal, look for how your nursing management could help you reach it.

IMPLEMENTATION AND MONITORING OF THE CHANGE STRATEGY

Now that you have identified your goal and developed your change strategy, you need to plan for monitoring your implementation process. Your action steps need to be evaluated for success and failure. When the planned action does not come to fruition or the action does not provide the results desired, new solutions need to be sought.

Effective evalutation is needed to decide what works and what does not work. Sometimes the action steps to reach the goal are unrealistic and the individual loses motivation because the goal seems unreachable. Steps are not meant to be leaps! Steps toward a goal need to be individually determined.

Trying to match someone else's steps is courting failure. Setting your action steps by considering your idiosyncrasies and establishing your own time line will lead you down the path to success. Most people unfortunately try to go about changing like most dieters do—they want it all now and set themselves up for the return of old habits by trying to change too quickly. Make sure your change steps are reasonable for you.

The more your evaluation is a consistent, ongoing process the more

Table 8-1
ASPECTS OF MONITORING YOUR CHANGE

1. Are your action steps reasonable?
2. Are your interim goals and rewards clear?
3. Are your steps individually determined?
4. Is your time line appropriate?
5. Is your monitoring system consistent and ongoing?
6. Are you prepared to treat setbacks as learning opportunities?
7. Are there at least two people with whom you will share your successes and setbacks?

likely you are to have reasonable steps. Adjustments in your change process are also important in minimizing the stress of change. By evaluating on an ongoing basis you will be able to detect the need for minor adjustments, thus averting major setbacks.

If setbacks occur due to inadequate planning or fate, it is important to remember to spend your time analyzing the problem, not beating yourself with guilt. Guilt, a feeling of inadequacy or hopelessness, destroys more change plans than fate. Going into any change process expecting a straight line of successes is bound to lead to disappointment.

Learning from your setbacks, developing consistent, ongoing evaluations, and setting up reasonable steps are the three aspects of monitoring your progress mentioned thus far. Two others are developing a reward system and utilizing your support system. Rewarding yourself as you achieve your interim goals fosters the feeling of achievement. List the rewards you will give to yourself at various points along the path of success. This pride in your accomplishment is meant to be shared. These successes can become resources that support achievement in more difficult goals.

The process outlined in this chapter is meant to act as a model for your changes. Answer the questions in Table 8-1 to check whether you have adequately planned for monitoring your proposed change.

If you answered "no" to any of these questions, go back and remedy the issue. If all your answers are "yeses," then you are ready to begin your change because your monitoring is established.

Remember that taking care of yourself is the most important task you have. Use this manual to refresh your memory as you progress with your stress management program. Best wishes for a successful and satisfying life.

References

Adams, J. D. Improving stress management: An action-research-based OD intervention. In W. W. Burke (Ed.), *The cutting edges.* San Diego: University Associates, 1978.

Adams, R. *The complete home guide to all the vitamins.* New York: Larchmont Books, 1978.

Adler, C. S., & Adler, S. M. Biofeedback-psychotherapy for the treatment of headaches: A 5-year follow-up. *Headache,* 1976, 189–191.

Aiken, L. Nursing priorities for the 1980's: Hospitals and nursing homes. *American Journal of Nursing,* 1981, 81, 325–330.

Albrecht, K. *Stress and the manager: Making it work for you.* Englewood Cliffs, N.J.: Prentice-Hall, 1979.

Allen, R. F. & Kraft, C. From burnout: Improving the quality of hospital work life. *Hospital Forum,* 1981, *24*(3), 18–28.

American Heart Association, *Standards for supervised cardiovascular exercise maintenance programs.* Dallas, Texas: May 1980.

American Hospital Association: *Eight and one-half percent differential suffers another assault by Feds. Hospitals,* 1981, *55*(2), 32, 35.

American Psychiatric Association. *Diagnostic and statistical manual of mental disorders* (4th edition), Washington, D.C., 1980.

Anderson, C. A., & Basteyns, M. Stress and critical care nurse reaffirmed. *Journal of Nursing Administration,* 1981, *11*, 31–34.

Anderson, R. The perfect pre-run stretching routine. *Runners World.* 1978, *13*, 56–61.

Ardell, D. B. *High level wellness: An alternative to doctors, drugs and disease.* Emmaus, Pa.: Rodale Press, 1977.

Arndt, C., & Huckabay, L. *Nursing administration: Theory for practice with a systems approach.* St. Louis: Mosby, 1980.

Arnold, J. D. *Make up your mind: The seven building blocks to better decisions.* New York: AMACOM, 1978.

Artz, T. The untapped health market. *Hospital Forum,* 1981, *24*, 21–26.

Averille, J. R. Personal control over aversive stimuli and its relationship to stress. *Psychological Bulletin,* 1973, *80*, 286–303.

Bailey, J. T. *Decision making in nursing: Roles for change.* St. Louis: Mosby, 1975.

Bailey, J. T., Steffen, S. M., & Grout, J. W. The stress audit: Identifying the stressors of ICU nursing. *Journal of Nursing Education,* 1980, *19*(5), 15–25.

Baker, D. The use and health consequences of shift work. *International Journal of Health Services,* 1980, *10*, 405–420.

Barnard, M. Closing the health care gap. *Kansas Medical Society,* 1974, *5*, 16–20.

Belfer, M. C., Shader, R. J., Carroll, M., & Harmatz, J. S. Alcoholism in women. *Archives of General Psychology.* 1971, *25*, 540–544.

Bell, J. M. Stressful life events and coping methods in mental-illness and wellness behaviors. *Nursing Research,* 1977, *26*, 136–141.

Benson, H. Yoga for drug abuse. *New England Journal of Medicine,* 1967, *281*, 1133.

Benson, H. Decreased systolic blood pressure in hypertensive subjects who practiced meditation. *Journal of Clinical Investigation,* 1973, *52*, 8a.

Benson, H. Decreased alcohol intake associated with the practice of meditation. A retrospective investigation. *Annals of the New York Academy of Sciences,* 1974, *233*, 174–177.

Benson, H., Rosner, B. A., Marzetta, B. R., & Klemchuk, H. M. Decreased blood pressure in borderline hypertensive subjects who practiced meditation. *Journal of Chronic Disease,* 1974, *27*, 163–169.

Benson, H. & Wallace, R. R. Decreased drug abuse with transcendental meditation. In J. D. Zeafonetis (Ed.), *Drug abuse—Proceedings of the international conference.* Philadelphia: Lea & Febiger, 1972, 369–376.

213

References

Bergson, A., & Tuchack, V. *Zone therapy.* New York: Pinnacle Books, 1974.

Berman, E. *The cooperating family: How your children can help manage the household for their good as well as yours.* Englewood Cliffs, N.J.: Prentice-Hall, 1977.

Beyer, J. E., & Marshall, J. The interpersonal dimension of collegiality. *Nursing Outlook,* 1981, *29,* 662–665.

Bissell, L. *Alcoholism and the health professional.* Paper presented at the Summer School in Alcoholic Studies, Rutgers University, June 27, 1979.

Bolton, R. *People skills.* Englewood Cliffs, N.J.: Prentice-Hall, 1979.

Brown, B. B. *New mind, new body.* New York: Harper & Row, 1974.

Burch, G. E., & Ansari, A. Chronic alcoholism and carcinoma of the pancreas: A correlative hypothesis. *Archives of Internal Medicine,* 1968, *122,* 273–275.

Budzynski, T. H., Stoyva, J. M., & Adler, C. S. Feedback induced muscle relaxation: Application to tension headache. *Journal of Behavioral Therapies and Experimental Psychiatry,* 1970, *1,* 205–211.

Buhler, C., & Massarik, F. (Eds.). *The course of human life: A study of goals in the humanistic perspective.* New York: Springer, 1968.

Burke, R. J. Occupational stress and job satisfaction. *Journal of Social Psychology,* 1976, *100,* 235–244.

Burns, D. D. *Feeling good: The new mood therapy.* New York: Signet Books, 1980.

Byrnes, M. A. Non-nursing functions: The nurses state their case. *American Journal of Nursing,* 1982, *82,* 1089–1097.

Cameron, N. Personality development and psychopathology: A dynamic approach. Boston: Houghton Mifflin, 1963.

Caplan, G. *Support system and community mental health.* New York: Behavioral Publications, 1974.

Cassem, N. H., & Hackett, T. P. Stress on the nurse and therapist in the intensive-care unit and coronary care unit. *Heart and Lung,* 1975, *4,* 252–259.

Clarke, H. *Physical fitness newsletter.* University of Oregon, Feb., 1979.

Claus, K., & Bailey, J. (Eds.). *Living with stress and promoting well being: A handbook for nurses.* St. Louis: Mosby, 1980.

Cleland, V. S. The effect of stress on performance. *Nursing Research,* 1965, *14,* 292–98.

Colen, B. D. The Valuim explosion: All things to all people. *Philadelphia Inquirer,* August 31, 1980.

Cooper, K. *The new aerobics.* New York: Bantam Books, 1970.

Cousins, N. *Anatomy of an illness as perceived by the patient: Reflections on healing and regeneration.* New York: Norton, 1979.

Conan, S. *Superwoman.* New York: Crown, 1978.

Cunningham, R. M. The trouble with nurses—They're human. *Hospitals,* 1981, *55*(23), 75–77.

Daley, M. R. Preventing worker burnout in child welfare. *Child Welfare,* 1979, *58,* 443–450.

Davis, A. *Let's eat right to keep fit.* New York: Harcourt Brace Jovanovich, 1954.

Davis, A. *Let's get well.* New York: Harcourt Brace Jovanovich, 1965.

Davis, M., Eshelman, E. R., & McKay, M. *The relaxation and stress reduction workbook.* Richmond, Calif.: New Harbinger, 1980.

Decreased federal spending threatens quality of care for elderly persons. *Hospitals,* 1981, *55*(2), 51–52.

Deluca, J. R. (Ed.). *Alcohol and health.* Rockville, Md.: National Institute on Alcohol Abuse and Alcoholism, 1981.

Dimock, M. *A philosophy of administration.* New York: Harper & Row, 1958.

Dodge, R. Operating to cut hospital costs. *Philadelphia Inquirer,* November 1, 1981.

Donovan, M. I. Study of the impact of relaxation with guided imagery on stress among cancer nurses. *Cancer Nursing,* 1981, *4,* 121–126.

Downing, G. *The massage book.* New York: Random House, 1972.

Drucker, P. F. *The effective executive.* New York: Harper & Row, 1967.

Drug Abuse Council. *Marijuana survey: State of Oregon.* January 28, 1977, Washington, D.C.

Duffy, W. *Sugar blues.* New York: Warner Communications, 1975.

Eisendrath, S. J., & Dunkel, J. Psychological issues in intensive care unit staff. *Heart and Lung,* 1979, *8,* 751–757.

Ellis, A., & Harper, R. *A new guide to rational living.* North Hollywood, Calif.: Wilshire Books, 1979.

Emener, W. G. Professional burnout: Rehabilitation's hidden handicap. *Journal of Rehabilitation,* 1979, *45,* 55–58.

Erikson, E. H. *Identity: Youth and crisis.* New York: W.W. Norton, 1968.

Ewald, E. B. *Recipes for a small planet.* New York: Balantine Books, 1973.

Fenner, L. Salt shakes up some of us (DHEW Publ. No. 80-2129). *Food and Drug Administration Consumer,* 1980, *3.*

Ferguson, T. The caffeine fix: It can cause many kinds of trouble. *Philadelphia Inquirer,* June 12, 1982.

Fiber: Not just for constipation any more. *Executive Fitness Newsletter,* 1980, *11*(4), 1–2.

Fiedler, F. *A theory of leadership effectiveness.* New York: McGraw-Hill, 1967.

Figler, H. E. *Path: A career workbook for liberal arts students.* Cranston, RI: Carroll Press, 1979.

Filley, A. C. *Interpersonal conflict resolution.* Glenview, Ill.: Scott, Foresman, 1975.

Florence Nightingale wants you! *Time,* August 24, 1981, 37.

Freud, A. *The Ego and the mechanisms of defense,* translated by C. M. Baines. New York: International Universities Press, 1956.

Freud, S. *The problem of anxiety.* New York: Norton, 1936.

Friedman, M. *Type A behavior and your heart.* Presentation at Sun Institute, Radnor, PA, April 1981.

Friedman, M., & Rosenman, R. *Type A behavior and your heart.* New York: Fawcett Books, 1974.

Gal, R., & Lazarus, R. S. The role of activity in anticipating and confronting stressful situations. *Journal of Human Stress,* 1975, *1*(4), 4–20.

Gank, S. Narcotic addiction in nurses and doctors. *Nursing Outlook,* 1975, *13*(11), 30–34.

Garb, S. Narcotic addiction in nurses and doctors. *Nursing Outlook,* 1965, *13,* 36–40.

Gardner, D., Parzen, Z. D., & Stewart, N. The nurses dilemma: Mediating stress in critical care units. *Heart and Lung,* 1980, *9,* 103–106.

Garfield, C. *Stress and survival: The emotional realities of life-threatening illness.* St. Louis: Mosby, 1979.

Gatchel, R. J., & Proctor, J. D. Physiological correlates of learned helplessness. *Journal of Abnormal Psychology, 1976, 85,* 27–34.

Gentry, W. D., Foster, S. B., & Froehling, M. S. Psychological response to situational stress in intensive and non-intensive nursing. *Heart and Lung,* 1972, 1, 793–796.

Goetz, A. A., Duff, J. F., & Bernstein, J. E. Health risk appraisal: Estimation of risk. *Public Health Reports,* 1980, *95,* 119–126.

Gordon, B. *I'm dancing as fast as I can.* New York: Bantam Books, 1979.

Gordon, G. G., & Southren, A. L. Metabolic effects of alcohol on the endocrine system. In C. S. Lieber (Ed.), *Metabolic aspects of alcoholism.* Baltimore: University Park Press, 1977, pp. 249–272.

Gordon, T. *Leader effectiveness training (L.E.T.): The no-lose way to release the productive potential of people.* New York: Wyden, 1977.

Gordon, T., & Burch, N. *T.E.T.: Teacher effectiveness training.* New York: Wyden, 1974.

Greene, W. A. The psychosocial setting of the development of leukemia and lymphoma. *Annals of the New York Academy of Sciences,* 1966, *125,* 794–801.

Hagnell, O. The premorbid personality of persons who develop cancer in a total population investigated in 1947 and 1957. *Annals of the New York Academy of Sciences,* 1966, *125,* 846–855.

Haley, J. (Ed.) *Advanced techniques of hypnosis and therapy: Selected papers of Milton Erickson.* New York: Grune & Stratton, 1967.

Hart, L.B. *Moving up! Moving up! Moving up! Women and leadership.* New York: AMACOM, 1980.

Hart, L. *Learning from conflict: A handbook for trainers and group leaders.* Reading, Mass.: Addison-Wesley, 1981.

Help for the helper. *American Journal of Nursing,* 1982, *82,* 572.

Hershey, P., & Blanchanrd, K. H. *Management of organizational behavior: Utilizing human resources,* (3rd ed.). Englewood Cliffs, N.J.: Prentice-Hall, 1977.

Herzburg, F., Mausner, B., & Sydernan, B. *The motivation to work.* (2nd ed.). New York: Wiley, 1959.

Hoffman, R. Stress and the critical care nurse. *Supervisor Nurse,* 1981, *12*(7), 20–23.

Holmes, T. H., & Rahe, R. H. The social readjustment rating scale. *Journal of Psychosomatic Research,* 1967, *11,* 213–218.

Horney, K. *Our inner conflicts.* New York: Norton, 1945.

Howe, R. *The miracle of dialogue.* New York: Seabury Press, 1963.

Huckabay, L., & Jagla, B. Nurses' stress factors in the intensive care unit. *Journal of Nursing Administration,* 1979, *9*(2), 21–26.

Hurst, M. W., Jenkins, C. D., & Rose, R. M. The relation of psychological stress to onset of medical illness. *Annual Review of Medicine,* 1976, *27,* 301–312.

Initial report and preliminary recommendations of the National Commission on Nursing. Chicago: American Hospital Association, 1981.

Isler, C. The alcoholic nurse: What we try to deny. *RN,* 1978, *41*(7), 48–55.

Ivancevich, J. M., & Matteson, M. T. Nurses and Stress: Time to examine the potential problem. *Supervisor Nurse,* 1980, *11*(6), 17–22.

Jacobson, E. *Progressive relaxation.* Chicago: The University of Chicago Press, Midway Report, 1974.

Jaffe, S. First-hand views of recovery. *American Journal of Nursing,* 1982, *82,* 578–579.

Janis, I. *Psychological stress.* New York: Wiley, 1958.

Jefferson, L. V., & Ensor, B. E. Confronting a chemically-impaired colleague. *American Journal of Nursing,* 1982, *82,* 574–577.

Jennings, E. An anatomy of leadership: Princes, heros and supermen. New York: McGraw-Hill, 1972.

Johnson, R. M., Richardson, J. I., Von Endt, L. L., & Lindgren, K. S. The professional support group: A model for psychiatric clinical nurse specialists. *Journal of Psychosocial Nursing and Mental Health Services,* 1982, *20*(2), 9–13.

Johnson, S. The health care crisis. *Working Woman,* September 1981, 84.

Johnson, S. H. Preventing group burnout. *Nursing Management,* 1982 *13*(2), 34–38.

Jones, J. W. *A measure of staff burnout among health professionals.* Paper presented at the annual national convention of the American Psychological Association, Montreal, Canada, 1980.

Jones, M. C. Personality antecedents and correlates of drinking patters in women. *Journal of Consulting and Clinical Psychology,* 1971, *36,* 61–69.

Kahn, R. L., Rosenthal, R. A. *Organizational stress: Studies in role conflict and role ambiguity.* New York: Wiley, 1964.

Kaltman, M. *Keeping up with keeping house: a practical guide for the harried housewife.* Garden City, N.Y.: Doubleday, 1971.

Karpman, S. B. Developments in transactional analysis. In J. H. Masserman (Ed.), *Current psychiatric therapies.* New York: Grune & Stratton, 1972.

Katz, C. A. Reducing interpersonal stress in dental practice. *Dental Clinics of North America,* 1978, *22,* 347–359.

Katz, D., & Kahn R. L. Some recent findings in human relations research in industry. In G. E. Swanson, T. M. Newcomb, & E. L. Hartley, *Readings in social psychology* (Rev. ed.). New York: Holt, 1952.

Katz, D., & Kahn, R. *The social psychology of organizations.* New York: Wiley, 1966.

Kaye, G. H., & Krol, S. The nursing shortage: This time traditional responses won't work. *Supervisor Nurse,* 1981, *12*(7), 13–17.

Keys, A. Diet and epidemiology of coronary heart disease. *Journal of the American Medical Association,* 1957, *164,* 1912.

Kinsey, B. A. *The female alcoholic: a social psychological study.* Springfield, Ill.: Thomas, 1966.

Kirschenbaum, H. *Beyond values clarification.* Upper Joy, N.Y.: National Humanistic Education Center, 1973.

Kirschenbaum, H. *Current research in values clarification.* Upper Joy, N.Y.: National Humanistic Education Center, 1975.

Kirschenbaum, H., & Glaser, B. *Developing support groups.* LaJolla, Calif.: University Associates, 1978.

Knaus, W. *Do it now: How to stop procrastinating.* Englewood Cliffs, N.J.: Prentice-Hall, 1979.

Knutzleman, C. *The Exerciser's Handbook.* New York: David McKay, 1978.

Knutzleman, C. T. *The complete book of walking.* New York: Pocket Books, 1982.

Kobasa, S. C., Hilker, R., & Maddi, S. R. Who stays healthy under stress? *Journal of Occupational Medicine,* 1979, *21,* 595–598.

Kraegal, J. M. *Organization–environment relationships.* Gaithersburg, MD.: Aspen Systems Corp., 1980.

Kramer, M., & Schmalenberg, C. *Path to biculturism.* Wakefield, Mass.: Nursing Resources, 1977.

Krantz, D. S. Cognitive processes and recovery from heart attack: A review and theoretical analysis. *Journal of Human Stress,* 1980, *6*(3), 27–38.

Kubler-Ross, E. *On death and dying.* New York: Macmillan, 1969.

Kubler-Ross, E. *Questions and answers on death and dying.* New York: Collier Books, 1974.

Lakein, A. *How to get control of your time and your life.* New York: Signet Books, 1973.

Lappe, F. M. *Diet for a small planet.* New York: Ballantine Books, 1975.

Lavendero, R. Nurse burnout: What can we learn? *Journal of Nursing Administration,* 1981, *11*(11–12), 17–23.

Lecos, C. Sugar: How sweet it is—And isn't (DHEW Publ. No. 80-2127). *Food and Drug Administration Consumer.* Rockville, MD: 1980, 2.

LeCron, L. *Self-hypnosis.* New York: New American Library, 1970.

LeShan, L. Psychological states as factors in the development of malignant disease: A critical review. *Journal of the National Cancer Institute,* 1959, *22,* 1–18.

LeShan, L. *How to meditate.* New York: Bantam Books, 1974.

LeShan, L., & Worthington, R. E. Loss of cathexis as a common psychodynamic characteristic of cancer patients. *Psychological Reports,* 1956, *2,* 83–193.

Lewin, K. *Field theory in social science.* New York: Harper, 1951.

Lewin, K., Lippit, R., & White, R. K. Patterns of aggressive behavior in experimentally created social climates. *Journal of Social Psychology,* 1939, *10,* 271–299.

Likert, R., & Likert, J. *New ways of managing conflict.* New York: McGraw-Hill, 1976.

Liman, E. *The spacemaker book.* New York: Viking Press, 1977.

Lindbeck, V. C. The woman alcoholic: A review of the literature. *International Journal of Addictions,* 1972, *7,* 567–580.

Lowen, A. *Bioenergetics.* New York: Penguin Books, 1976.

Lyons, T. F. Role clarity, need for clarity, satisfaction, tension, and withdrawal. *Organizational Behavior and Human Performance,* 1971, *6,* 99–110.

Maaksel, I. *Future of nursing.* Presentation at continuing education event of Pennsylvania Nurses' Association, Mt. Airy, PA, 1979.

Machlowitz, M. M. *Workaholics: Living with them, working with them.* Reading, Mass.: Addison-Wesley, 1980.

Magula, M. *Understanding organizations: A guide for the nurse executive.* Gaithersburg, MD: Aspen Systems Corp., 1982.

Marram, G. D. *The group approach in nursing practice.* St. Louis: Mosby, 1973.

Martin, A. A., & Tenenbaum, F. *Diet against disease: A new plan for safe and healthy eating.* Boston: Houghton Mifflin, 1980.

May, R. *The meaning of anxiety.* New York: Roland, 1950.

McCarty, P. Hospitals share success stories. The *American Nurse,* 1982, *14*(5), 1, 7, 17.

McKenna, J. F., Oritt, P. L., & Wolff, H. K. Occupational stress as a prediction in the turnover decision. *Journal of Human Stress,* 1981, *7*(4), 12–17.

Merzen, M. *Winning the diet wars.* New York: Harcourt Brace Jovanovich, 1980.

Meyer, P. J. *The dynamics of personal leadership.* Waco, Tex.: Success Motivation Institute, 1976.

Miller, G. P. *Life choices: How to make the critical decisions about your education, career, marriage, family and lifestyle.* New York: Crowell, 1978.

Mirin, S. N., Shapiro, L. M, Meyer, R. E., Pillard, R. C., & Fisher, S. Casual versus heavy use of marijuana: A redefinition of the marijuana problem. *American Journal of Psychiatry,* 1971, *127,* 54–60.

Morris, F. *Self-hypnosis in two days.* Berkeley, Calif.: Intergalactic, 1974.

Mott, P. E. Social and psychological adjustment to shift work. In *Shift work and health (DHEW Publ. No. 76-203).* Washington, D.C.: U.S. Department of Health, Education, and Welfare, 1976.

Muktananda, S. *Where are you going?: A guide to the spiritual journey.* Ganeshpuri, India: Gurudeva Siddha Path, 1981.

Mundinger, M. *Autonomy in nursing.* Gaithersburg, Md.: Aspen Systems Corp. 1980.

Munro, J. D. Preventing front-line collapse in institutional settings. *Hospital and Community Psychiatry,* 1980, *31,* 179–182.

Murray, R. M. Psychiatric illnesses in doctors. *Lancet,* 1974, 1, 1211–1213.

Naranjo, C., & Ornstein, R. *The psychology of meditation.* New York: Viking Press, 1971.

National Academy of Sciences. *Marijuana and health and analysis of marijuana policy.* Washington, D.C., June, 1982.

National Cancer Institute (NIH publication No. 8101647). *Clearing the air: A guide to quitting smoking.* Bethesda, MD: National Institutes of Health, 1981.

National Cancer Institute. *Why do you smoke?* (NIH Publ. No. 80-1822). Bethesda, MD: National Institutes of Health, 1980.

National Clearing House for Drug Abuse. *Stimulants: Some questions and some answers* (DHEW Publ. No. HSM-71-9026). Washington, D.C.: U.S. Government Printing Office, 1981.

National Institute on Drug Abuse. *National survey of drug abuse.* Rockville, Md.: 1979.

Nyswander, M. Drug addictions. In S. Arieti (Ed.), *American handbook of psychiatry*. New York: Basic Books, 1959, 614–622.

O'Conner, A. B. (Ed.). *Dying and grief: Nursing intervention* (Contemporary Nursing Series). New York: American Journal of Nursing, 1976.

Odiorne, G. *Management by objectives*. New York: Pitman, 1965.

Odiorne, G. Management by objectives: Antidote to future shock. *Journal of Nursing Administration*, 1975, *5*, 27–30.

Orbach, S. *Fat is a feminist issue*. New York: Berkley Books, 1978.

Oskins, S. L. Identification of situational stressors and coping methods by intensive care nurses. *Heart and Lung*, 1979, *8*, 953–960.

Pelletier, K. *Mind as healer, mind as slayer: A holistic approach to preventing stress disorders*. New York: Delta Book, 1977.

Pines, A. Burnout: A current problem in pediatrics. *Current Problems in Pediatrics*, 1981, *11*, 1–32.

Pines, A., & Aronson, E. *Burnout: From tedium to personal growth*. New York: Free Press, 1981.

Pines, A., & Kafry, D. Occupational teduim in the social services. *Social Work*, 1978, *23*, 499–507.

Pines, A., & Maslach, C. Characteristics of staff burnout in mental health settings. *Hospital and Community Psychiatry*, 1978, 29, 233–237.

Polak, M. The search for life after Valium. *Philadelphia Inquirer Today Magazine*, November 1, 1981.

Poplar, J. F. Characteristics of nurse addicts. *American Journal of Nursing*, 1969, *69*, 117–119.

Ramprasad, G. Evaluation of stress in non-manual work: An empirical investigation. *Indian Journal of Medical Research*, 1973, *61*, 1714, 1721.

Rolf, I. P. *Rolfing: The integration of the human structure*. Santa Monica, Calif.: Dennis-Landman, 1977.

Rosa, K. *You and AT: Autogenic training*. New York: Dutton, 1973.

Russell, C. Fitness fetish. *American Demographics*, 1980, *2*(10), 40–41.

Schachter, S. Alkaline-acid effect on smokers. *Journal of Behavioral Ecology*, 2(2), 1981.

Schiff, J. *Cathexis reader: Transactional analysis treatment of psychosis*. New York: Harper & Row, 1975.

Selye, H. *Stress without distress*. New York: Signet Books, 1974.

Selye, H. *The stress of life*. New York: McGraw-Hill, 1976.

Shaw, M. E. A comparison of two types of leadership in various communication nets. *Journal of Abnormal Psychology*, 1955, *50*, 127–134.

Shealy, N. *Ninety days to self-health*. New York: Bantam Books, 1977.

Signs and symptoms of the alcoholic nurse. Columbus, Ohio: Ohio Nurses Association Peer Assistance Program for Nurses, 1981.

Signs and symptoms of the drug addicted nurse. Columbus, Ohio: Ohio Nurses Association Peer Assistance Program for Nurses, 1981.

Simon, S. B., Howe, L. W., & Kirschenbaum, H. *Values clarification: A handbook of strategies for teachers and students*. New York: Hart, 1972.

Skelsey, A. *The working mother's guide to her home, her family and herself*. New York: Random House, 1970.

Spreads, C. *Breathing—The ABC's*. New York: Harper & Row, 1978.

Stehle, J. L. Critical care nursing stress: The findings revisited. *Nursing Research*, 1981, 30, 182–186.

Stevens, B. J. *The nurse as executive*. Gaithersburg, Md.: Aspen Systems Corp., 1980.

Stieglitz, H. Concepts of organization planning. In H. E. Frank (Ed.)., *Organizing structuring*. New York: McGraw-Hill, 1971.

References

Strahinich, J. Endorphin Puzzle. *The Runner,* 1982, *7,* 48–50.

Study tracking stress response. *Training: Magazine of Human Resources Development,* 1981, *18*(6), 87.

Suls, J., & Mullen, B. Life events, Perceived control and illness. *Journal of Human Stress,* 1981, *7*(2), 30–34.

Sutterly, D., & Donnelly, G. (Eds.). *Coping with stress: A nursing perspective.* Gaitersburg, Md.: Aspen Systems Corp., 1982.

Tasto, D., Colligan, M., Skjen, E., & Polly, S. Health consequences of shift work (DHEW Publ. No. 75–154). Washington, D.C.: U.S. Department of Health, Education and Welfare, U.S. Government Printing Office, 1978.

Tennov, D. *Superself: A woman's guide to self-management.* New York: Funk & Wagnalls, 1977.

Thomas, C. B., & Greenstreet, R. L. Psychological characteristics in youth as predictors of five disease states: Suicide, mental illness, hypertension, coronary heart disease, and tumor. *John Hopkins Medical Journal,* 1973, *132,* 16–43.

U.S. Department of Health, Education, and Welfare. *Marijuana and health* (DHEW Publ. No. 72-9113). Washington, D.C.: U.S. Government Printing Office, 1972.

U.S. Department of Health, Education, and Welfare. *Shift work* (DHEW Publ. No. 76-203). Washington, D.C.: U.S. Government Printing Office, 1976.

U.S. Senate Select Committee on Nutrition and Human Needs. *Dietary goals for the United States.* Washington, D.C.: U.S. Government Printing Office, 1977.

Valliant, G. Health consequences of adaptations of life. *The American Journal of Medicine,* 1979, *67,* 732–734.

Veninga, R. Administration burnout—Causes and cures. *Hospital Progress,* 1979, *60*(2), 45–52.

Veninga. R. L. Work, stress and health: Four major conclusions. *Occupational Health Nursing,* 1982, *30*(6), 22–24.

Vreeland, R., & Ellis, G. Stresses of the nurse in an intensive care unit. *Journal of the American Medical Association,* 1969, *208,* 332–334.

Wandelt, M., Hales, G. D., Merwin, C. M., Olsson, N. G. Pierce, P. M., & Widdowson, R. R. *Conditions associated with registered nurse employment in Texas.* Austin: The University of Texas at Austin School of Nursing, 1980.

What the SNA's are doing in Maryland, Georgia, Ohio, and Tennessee. *American Journal of Nursing,* 1982, *82,* 581–585.

Wheelan, S. *The planned change model of personal growth.* Philadelphia: PEP Center Monograph Series of Temple University, 1978.

Wiekramaskekera, I. Electromyographic feedback training and tension headache: Preliminary observations. *American Journal of Clinical Hypnosis,* 1972, *15,* 83–85.

Wikler, A. *Opiate addiction.* Springfield, Ill.: Thomas, 1953.

Winston, S. *Getting organized. The easy way to put your life in order.* New York: Warner Books, 1978.

Work conditions cause nurses to leave. *The American Nurse,* 1980, *12*(10), 5, 19.

Zander, A. *Groups at work: Unresolved issues in the study of organizations.* San Francisco: Jossey-Bass, 1977.

Zander, K. S. *Primary nursing: Development and management.* Gaithersburg, Md.: Aspen Systems Corp., 1980.

Zinberg, N. E. The war over marijuana. *Psychology Today,* 1976, *10*(7), 45–52, 102, 106.

Zindler-Wernet, P., & Bailey, J. T. Coping with stress through an "on-site" running program for Stanford ICU nurses. *Journal of Nursing Education,* 1980, *9*(6), 34–37.

Index